The Poetics of Sleep

Also Available From Bloomsbury

The Poetics of Sleep
From Aristotle to Nancy

Simon Morgan Wortham

B L O O M S B U R Y

LONDON • NEW DELHI • NEW YORK • SYDNEY

Bloomsbury Academic

An imprint of Bloomsbury Publishing Plc

50 Bedford Square	175 Fifth Avenue
London	New York
WC1B 3DP	NY 10010
UK	USA

www.bloomsbury.com

First published 2013

British Library Cataloguing-in-Publication Data
A catalogue record for this book is available from the British Library.

ISBN: HB: 978-1-4411-2476-0
ePub: 978-1-4411-8081-0
ePDF: 978-1-4411-6962-4

Library of Congress Cataloging-in-Publication Data
Wortham, Simon.
The poetics of sleep : from Aristotle to Nancy / Simon Morgan Wortham.
p. cm.
Includes bibliographical references (p.   ) and index.
ISBN 978-1-4411-2476-0 (hardcover)– ISBN 978-1-4411-6962-4 (ebook pdf)– ISBN 978-1-4411-8081-0 (epub) 1. Sleep. 2. Dreams. I. Title.
BF1071.W67 2013
128'.4--dc23
2012028312

Typeset by Fakenham Prepress Solutions, Fakenham, Norfolk NR21 8NN
Printed and bound in Great Britain

Contents

Acknowledgements

My thanks are due to Sarah Campbell for her encouragement and support in all aspects of this project, and to Camilla Erskine for her assistance in its final stages. 'The entire mental life minus the effort of concentration' – Bergson's definition of dreaming – probably applies equally to Martin McQuillan's contribution to this volume. Thanks finally to Ceri, who once called me a bulimic sleeper, for surviving another book. This one's for you.

Introduction: The Poetics of Sleep

You might as well be dead/dreaming's black box

In his 1977 book *The Sleep Instinct*, the psychologist Ray Meddis advances the theory (one he had held for over a decade by that time) that 'sleep serves no important function in modern man and that, in principle at least, man is capable of living happily without it'.[1] Sleep evolved, so the argument goes, not as a means for living creatures to achieve vital rest after physical and mental exertion, in order to overcome fatigue, or to recuperate and revive, but as a way to maximize the chances of survival during those long periods, once the hunt for food and other basic tasks are over, when animals really have nothing else to do. Sleep is thus essentially a 'spare-time activity' (p. 14) which converts unavoidable inertia or idleness into a means of self-protection. Sleep, often thought of as a state of vulnerability, in fact keeps living creatures out of trouble. It renders them inconspicuous. It usually keeps them out of sight or at any rate leads them to a safe place. It keeps them still and thus ensures immobility and therefore non-responsiveness to external stimuli as a key safety-mechanism, and so on. Accordingly, notes Meddis, if one observes the sleep-patterns of animals in a variety of natural settings, it can be seen that, for the most part, 'sleep expands and contracts in keeping with the available spare time' enjoyed by each species (p. 24). Indeed, for Meddis, wide discrepancies in the ratio of wakefulness to sleep found in different species (and, for that matter, within them – particularly among humans) supports his view that sleep cannot simply be a restorative activity, just a matter of recuperation or system-repair.[2]

As a survival-technique rather than a repair-tool, however, sleep for 'modern man' seems somewhat redundant, a mere hangover from evolutionary history. Preserving us from dangers that are now, by and large, ancient ghosts (or that we have found other, more sophisticated ways to fend off), human sleep is really little more than an enjoyable ritual (like non-reproductive sex) that has become hard-wired into the brain, as its 'sleep-control mechanism' – supported by a 'powerful central-nervous-system mechanism which induces feelings of drowsiness' (p. 12) – creates sleep-motives 'which make sleep-related achieve-ments more pleasurable and other achievements less so' (p. 4). (Meddis tells us that 'drowsiness increases according to a plan or stratagem whose aim is to get you to bed' (p. 11).) If only we could find a way to adjust the circuitry of the human brain, with its long-evolved 'sleep stat', much wasted time could be avoided. 'It may require a brain operation or more hopefully a simple injection', Meddis speculates, but thankfully that may not be too far into the future. 'We shall have to wait and see', he prudently adds, although only after insisting rather more darkly that we can indeed 'expect' the scientific knowledge and techno-logical means necessary for brain-adjustment to be 'available soon' (p. 32). (At the present time, Meddis laments, we have to rely on accidental brain injuries to provide scientific information about all of this; although he also fantasizes about the possibility of luring a fabled 'nonsomniac' into the laboratory, 'where proper checks and measurements can be made' (p. 37).[3]) Faced with the prospect of deliberately re-tuning the brain, some may have certain reservations, needless to say; but, early on in the book at any rate, Meddis seems to feel sure the prize would be well worth the winning.[4] As he rather grandly puts it, 'sleep has important non-recuperative functions in animals which may no longer apply to civilised man' (p. i): if evolution will prove too slow in fixing things, surely the 'civilised' thing to do would be to take a hand ourselves?

Now compare Plato's commentary on sleep, more than two millennia earlier (close to what Meddis may presume to be the dawn of civilization itself). Plato is in the midst of writing that 'every gentleman must have a timetable prescribing what he is to do every minute of his life, which he should follow at all times from the dawn of one day until the sun comes up at the dawn of the next'.[5] While, as he recognizes, the law – if it is to retain its dignity – cannot be expected to micro-manage personal timetables, never-theless a genuine need arises to curtail sleep at night, whether by legal means or simply by custom. This is necessary in the interests of protecting the 'entire state', 'systematically and uninterruptedly', as the English translation puts it. Sleeping a whole night through is therefore simply a disgrace for a gentleman, who should make a point of being the first in the household to rise, long before his servants (and he should be *seen* to do so). In addition, Plato insists, 'while awake at night, all citizens should transact a good proportion of their political and domestic business, the officials up and down the town, masters and mistresses in their private households'. Physical and mental alertness and activity are not only virtues in their own right, they serve to confirm and support the seamless continuity and ever-presence of the life of the state in all its constituent parts, public and private, official and domestic (a state, that is, continually buzzing like the networks of a hyperactive, hyper-dynamic brain, an unstintingly vital cerebrum on a vast scale). More ominously, perhaps, ever-alert officials, wide awake at night, 'inspire fear in the wicked, whether citizens or enemies', while in the 'just' and 'virtuous' they instil 'courage' and emulous admiration. The good citizen, then, also wakes early, to send their children off to school. 'Children must not be left without teachers', writes Plato, 'nor slaves without masters' – the two presumably going hand in hand. 'Asleep,' concludes Plato, 'a man is useless, he may as well be dead.' (This would only seem to confirm Meddis's hunch that the risks of brain surgery in the interests of sleep-adjustment are well worth it in the end. Be that as it may, on several occasions throughout this book we will have cause to come back to this implied connection between sleep and death.)

Now, I do not draw attention to this passage from Plato merely to observe that any study of the natural advantages of sleep-behaviour would benefit from a further inquiry into the organizational and disciplinary *politics* of sleep[6] in a variety of 'states' or communities which may, in fact, not merely be limited to the 'human' (obviously while Meddis argues that sleep extends to fill the available spare-time in the lower life-forms of the 'animal kingdom', Plato makes crystal clear exactly *why* it should be characteristic of 'civilized' human life that this tendency is reversed, forcibly if necessary). Nor is my aim simply to ridicule and undermine Meddis's theory of sleep by showing how it replays age-old assumptions about the fatuousness and unseemliness of prolonged slumber in 'civilized' man, derived as these assumptions may be from a sort of classical fascism. My larger point is this: sometimes at the very moment they claim to break new ground or depart from conventional thinking, developing theories and trends in sleep science – for good or ill, unwittingly or not – may draw upon the long-standing and often occluded resources of the philosophical canon.[7] (In his Preface, perhaps unsurprisingly, Meddis tells us very confidently that his theory swims against the 'mainstream', opposes 'established orthodoxy', countering both 'current medical thought' and plain 'common sense'.)

Despite its odd mixture of the quirky (as we might euphemistically say) and the surprisingly predictable, Meddis's thesis does something very interesting to the physiological explanation for sleep, one that often prevails even throughout theories of dreaming (which themselves have frequently tended to characterize dreams as an expression of the life of the 'mind' in contradistinction to sleep as a purely physiological matter, certainly over much of the long period covered by this book). For his argument at once asserts that sleep evolved as a way to preserve physical life, though as a form of *behaviour* (rather than a 'natural' need), while at the same time arguing for its non-necessity (or at any rate its secondary importance) as a repair-mechanism working on behalf of such 'physical' preservation. Throughout this book, we will come back to the question of how physiological explanations of sleep have worked, what their indebtedness to the philosophical tradition may be, and how they may serve to complicate and confound as much as enable certain forms of thought or inquiry which concern themselves with sleep. To the extent that Meddis pursues his theory by engaging with the science of the brain, however, he profoundly questions the belief that sleep occurs so that the brain may simply *rest*. In fact, this echoes a general view among sleep scientists of the past few decades that brain activity is not merely switched-off, suspended, lowered or reduced during sleep, but rather that the brain is activated differently during different periods or types of slumber.[8] 'So far, everything we have learnt about the brain indicates that it could continue indefinitely, like the heart, without any pause for refuelling', Meddis writes (p. 6). (Indeed, for Meddis, sleep is not a blanket state of total unconsciousness but, more properly observed, it mainly puts living creatures into various states of *semi*-consciousness, whereby they in fact remain alert and responsive to some stimuli but not others: for instance, we may awaken upon hearing our name called, or the sound of an alarm, but sleep on through an equally noisy burst of birdsong or the revving of a car engine.[9]) While considering dreams, meanwhile, Meddis writes that 'the major piece of evidence, supporting the basic idea that dreams are necessary for sanity, has now gone and dream-repair theories remain as much a matter of faith as they have always been' (p. 70). Although Meddis does acknowledge that dreams may serve a useful function in such things as memory reorganization, more generally he extends to dreaming his deep-seated rejection of the idea of sleep as something restorative, denying there is convincing evidence that dreams are required to re-establish some sort of psychic equilibrium as a counterpart to physiological rest and recuperation. Instead, by way of a quite technical scientific argument, he proposes that dreaming can be understood as entirely consistent with the 'immobilization theory' of sleep he proposes, rather than the 'repair theory' he wants to falsify. Thus, he argues, dreams as much as sleep are not about psychic or physiological 'rest', either for the body or the brain. Once more, this resonates with other perspectives in the science of sleep which question the idea that dreaming functions foremost to address unresolved or suppressed psychic material. For instance, J. Allan Hobson argues that 'it is already crystal clear that many aspects of dreaming previously thought to be meaningful, privileged and interpretable psychologically are the simple reflection of the sleep-related changes in the brain'.[10] For Hobson, the Freudian conception of dreaming as a psychological reaction to the unconscious (in particular, to repressed or censored wishes) is strongly challenged by the results produced by electroencephalographic testing, which support the idea of selective alterations in brain chemistry and circuitry being responsible for the formal properties of dreams (for example, dreaming during REM sleep as dramatic, complex, bizarre, hallucinatory, delusional, irrational, incongruous, emotionally intense, and so forth). For Hobson, then, what happens during sleep and dreaming is largely explicable in terms of changes to the brain's 'mode of operation' by a chemical alteration and 'selective brain deactivation' which nonetheless serves to heighten or enhance some mental functions in the process of reducing others (p. 12).[11] (As he insists, 'the brain is always more active than not' (p. 161).) Hence, the psychological interpretation of dreaming – and especially the psychoanalytic emphasis on repression, censorship, or 'disguise', as Hobson puts it – is by and large mistaken and misguided, since dreams have little intrinsic 'psychological' function or meaning, but are instead mainly the trivial by-products of such electro-chemical processes in brain activity or neurophysiology (which is continuous but simply varies between sleep and wakefulness – implying that the waking 'mind' is, like dreaming, just an epiphenomenon of neurobiology). Hobson suggests that, during sleep, vital aspects of our cognitive ability – those which organize our memories in order to aid survival – may be strengthened and restored as an important feature of brain function (here, he seems to depart somewhat from his own emphasis on dreaming as just an epiphenomenon of brain activity); nonetheless, Hobson's argument does not rely on a simple idea of the brain as at *rest* during slumber.

While we are on the subject, it is worth pointing out that the function of dreams, if there is any, still remains a matter of great theoretical debate among neuroscientists studying sleep. D. Kuiken has recently summarized the main avenues of inquiry concerning dreaming, arguing that they may not be simply contradictory or competing in their claims, but might in future be integrated into a combined approach appropriate to different aspects of sleep:

> Perhaps the most common proposal is that dreams metaphorically represent disturbing life events and allow the covert review of self-protective or self-restorative processes. Another long-standing hypothesis is that dreaming distinctively reorganises memories for newly learned tasks and enhances the retrieval of related knowledge and skills ... another conception is that dreaming directly alters attention, evokes feeling, and enhances the flexibility and emotional relevance of postdream thought.[12]

Despite this eloquent summary of key approaches, however, the editors of the volume in which Kuiken writes assert in their Preface that, setting aside the continuing lack of detailed knowledge about many sleep-functions, 'dreaming is still almost as obscure a black box as it was half a century ago'. Which is to say, around the time REM sleep was discovered, in 1953. In fact, this was in the same year as the discovery of the structure of DNA, which as they point out has 'led to the development of the entire field of molecular biology and spawned the biotechnology industry' – achievements hardly matched by advances in sleep research. Indeed, in the same Preface, differences in emphasis once again suggest themselves at the point we are warned not to treat sleep as principally a 'physiological state', but to understand it more subtly and complexly as in fact 'a state of consciousness'.[13] (Several times throughout this book, we will ask about the *inter-implication* of notions of 'physiology' and of 'consciousness' in various forms of thinking about sleep and dreaming.)

But let's get back to Meddis. For all the self-assurance that underlies his thesis, its two central convictions, when combined, leave us in a somewhat uncertain situation. For while the falsely supposed 'need' to sleep should be actively conquered by the waking mind (both that of the clear-headed scientist and the civilized 'modern man'), it turns out that, in any case, far from ceasing to be active during sleep, the brain is – as Hobson and others would concur – as dynamic and functional as ever during slumber, and simply involved in a different order of activity. One might wonder if there isn't a certain sort of kettle logic at work here: why resist the inactivity or immobility brought on by sleep if it is in fact, and in principle, the expression of neurological activity that is just as 'active' as that of the waking brain? The answer, of course, has to do with consciousness, or at any rate a particular conception of consciousness. It has to do with the idea that – despite the many advances, insights and re-orientations of neurological science – the activity associated with the 'waking mind' is still to be set at a different level of priority and value than that of the 'sleeping' brain (even in a theoretical work, like Meddis's, that claims to banish old prejudices and instead to welcome the latest neuro-scientific discoveries and innovations).

From Aristotle to Nancy

In the first chapter of this book, we will therefore begin by looking at the question of sleep's relation to 'sense-perception' and 'consciousness' in Aristotle and indeed in the contested legacy of reading Aristotle, which is of course highly significant for the avenues philosophy will have taken over the past two millenia. In some ways, Aristotle seems to argue that sleep is mainly a physiological response to the natural demands or workings of the body. However, he also suggests that sleep arises as an expression or condition of the organ of sense-perception, which is itself the sign of the soul's transport through the body. It may well be that these two emphases, far from being simply antithetical to one another, give rise to complex interactions in the thinking of physiology and consciousness over time, interactions that we need to attend to in their specific and singular manifestations. As Derrida points out, however, the question of sleep also becomes important to the way in which Heidegger explores the possibility of a different reading of Aristotle than the one which simply positions him as a crucial reference point in thinking about the classical antecedents for a modern conception of consciousness.

Jumping ahead to the Enlightenment, the chapter explores the implications of Kant's idea that sleep entails a 'relaxation' which is also simultaneously a 'gathering of power for renewed external sensations',[14] albeit one that (in accord, perhaps, with Plato's instructions) should be taken in proper measure, as a functional expression and productive supplement of rational, waking life. (Here, the figure of the somnambulist, which in fact recurs with relative frequency throughout the 'text' of philosophy, proves troubling for Kant.) Thus sleep supports life, which is in fact defended by dreaming, since by stirring us – not least, in times of danger – dreams prevent sleep from leading towards or turning into death. Dreams, in other words, become the necessary adjunct or, as Freud would later put it, the 'guardians' of sleep, saving sleep from itself, stopping it from becoming total and thus deathly. The idea of dreaming as the sleep-resistant core at the heart of sleep itself undoubtedly involves complexities that Kant does not seek or want to grasp fully. Indeed, since sleeping and dreaming are principally to be thought of as instruments serving the interests of waking life, their misuse, misapplication or misappropriation makes possible certain dangers – sleep-walking, irrational conduct, delusion, and a propensity to excessive sleep which may, Kant suggests, give rise to premature death. Such perils are in one sense destined precisely due to the conceptual restriction of sleep – as that which is more truly auto-immune (having to resist itself) – to its mere 'functionality'.

In Hegel, meanwhile, dreams do not so much prise open the entire spectrum of the mind's workings, in comparison to the more restricted or 'concentrated' perceptions associated with wakefulness (as Bergson would have it), but instead they are simply what happens to perception when the self as a 'totality for itself' somewhat loses hold. Relatedly, for Hegel, the withdrawal-into-itself of the 'soul' that happens during sleepwalking, since it comes at the price of excluding 'the power of *mental* consciousness' (as Hegel puts it), far from leads to the felicitous (re)integration of being. Rather, the utter abandonment of the 'soul' to itself militates against being-for-self, since by sacrificing what Hegel calls 'the objective relation to the actual world' the self risks not only its reason but its unity and cohesiveness as such. Indeed, in the Hegelian 'text' an implied menace lurks deep in the heart of sleep. For the withdrawal into itself of the 'soul' in deepest slumber looks to be inescapable – at any rate, it is a need which the mind seems to have – and yet at the same time such a withdrawal establishes the grounds for the disorder of somnambulism. Put differently, Hegel's own argument suggests the idea that illness or disorder may be due to an inherent imbalance in sleep. His subsequent attempts to reassert '*mental* consciousness' over the forces which threaten it (which in turn involves giving the 'soul' a more positive slant in terms of its relationship to being-for-self) thus call for attentive reading. In fact, Hegel somewhat shifts position in order to suggest that the being-for-self which hitherto had been represented in terms of the priority of '*mental* consciousness' over the impending disorder of the 'soul' should in fact be understood in terms of a less oppositional connection between the two, and a more integrated mutuality. However, to the extent that it is dialectical thought which arranges, more or less surreptitiously, for the re-elevation of the previously dominant term, precisely by way of this apparent synthesis, the motivation underlying such a seeming change in reasoning is of enormous interest. More generally, then, the chapter suggests that, throughout these selections from the philosophical canon, a strange effect occurs, one with which all subsequent thought must grapple. For, in the process of treating sleep as ultimately integrated with the interests of both bodily and waking life, something else is let loose (somnambulance would be just one name for it), something which cannot be incorporated, excluded, or downplayed without trouble.

In the following chapter, we begin by contrasting Bergson's work on sleep and dreaming to that of Freud. (Bergson's essay 'Dreams' appeared about the same time as *The Interpretation of Dreams*, around the turn of the twentieth century.) For Bergson, the explanation for dreams lies not in the workings of the 'unconscious' but instead arises from the specific interaction of memory and sensation in a dreaming mind characterized by a form of perception that is unrestricted by the probabilistic interpretation of reality which typifies wakefulness. Thus dreaming is just 'the entire mental life minus the effort of concentration', as he famously puts it. Since, despite this difference, dreams are basically 'elaborated almost in the same way as perception of the real world' (to quote Bergson), Bergsonian thought resonates in certain respects with the neuro-scientific claim that what happens during sleep is not simply a matter of pure physiology outside consciousness, but has do with an alternate state of 'consciousness' that in turn puts in question what we might mean by the term itself. In his thinking about dreams, of course, Freud chooses the 'royal road' of the unconscious. For Freud, as yet unprocessed stimuli from the outside world, or in other words the residues of the day, are merely the 'entrepreneur' unleashing the potent 'capital' of unconscious wishes. Thus day-time remainders are, relatively speaking, 'trifling' in importance when interpreting dreams. And yet dreaming is not purely 'somatic', as Freud force-fully argues: to the extent that the material dealt with in dreams relates to unconscious wishes that are predominantly infantile in terms of their prove-nance, dreams do not just come from the night-time, nor is their meaning or impact restricted to it. The complex and ambivalent relationship of sleep and dreaming to 'day' in its double sense therefore sets the scene for an interplay between wakefulness and slumber which remains difficult to resolve. From this, I argue, sleep is radically double-facing in Freud's work. It serves the conscious wish to sleep and the workings of the unconscious at once, since the ability to hold down repressed material is reduced by a certain, unavoidable relaxation of energy during sleep, while at the same time dreaming expends unused energy or 'interest' in a way that is 'innocuous' to sleep, allowing the slumberer to dream on without awakening. The difficulty of knowing in which or in whose *interests* one sleeps therefore unsettles the idea of sleep as a crudely physiological matter (the notion of sleep as an inert substrate or mere platform is left without *basis* at the point where sleep's 'interests' remain undecided), while also disrupting the conception of sleep and dreaming as ultimately the expression of a 'consciousness' (as conventionally construed). In Freud's 'A Metaphysical Supplement to the Theory of Dreams', meanwhile, the doubleness of sleep takes on a particular hue. Here, dreaming is not just a means of wallowing in the deep narcissism shared by the ego and the libido alike, as Freud elsewhere sought to argue. It is also a matter of tackling those unresolved psychic residues that threaten to break into and disturb the narcis-sistic dream. Crucially, this threat to the narcissistic indulgence of dreaming which comes from day-time remainders isn't just a matter of *external* menace, because for Freud such residues acquire significance precisely to the extent that they retain a certain degree of *libidinal* 'interest'. Thus, I argue, the dream sees narcissism defending itself against what are basically its *own* interests. For Freud, in fact, this may be what a dream is. Perhaps it is no surprise, then, that in his essay 'On Narcissism' Freud presents sleep as similar to illness and yet, by way of the same analogy, also a means of defence against sickness. This prompts us to ask whether it is because narcissism is basically *auto-immune* that the sleep which ostensibly serves and supports it is at once a matter of illness and health, well-being and malady, ailment and cure. Does the double-facing nature of sleep tell us something about the way in which narcissism takes 'exception' to itself (as Freud himself implies it does)? As I argue, Freud's apparent U-turn regarding the narcissism of the ego/libido in sleep (whereby both end up in an allergic reaction to sleep) forms part of a highly volatile reaction to the auto-immune condition of narcissism itself; a reaction in which Freud's own text participates. What might be the future of such Freudian sleep? The chapter concludes with a consideration of this question, via a reading of Jacqueline Rose's essay, 'On Not Being Able to Sleep'.

As we shall see, Jean-Luc Nancy has recently insisted: 'There is no phenomenology of sleep'. Be that as it may, Chapter 3 looks to the work of Husserl and Merleau-Ponty. In Husserl, time-consciousness involves a retentional consciousness of that which may have elapsed but nonetheless remains essential in its sequencing with, or of, the present. The difference between 'near' and 'far' retention – the just-past and the long-since – is described by Husserl in terms of the distinction between 'falling asleep' and 'being asleep'. Since, as Nicolas de Warren has recently observed, such falling-asleep of consciousness as a type of 'self-forgetting' is intrinsic to how time-consciousness constitutes itself, it is possible to argue that in Husserl a certain sleep in fact makes possible wakefulness or consciousness itself. For Merleau-Ponty, meanwhile, the structure of perception is not based purely in 'consciousness' construed in terms of the disembodied mind, but is rather that of an 'emotional totality' in which the 'subject' is integrated and included along with the 'object' of perception, as a basic condition of perception's possibility. Thus perception depends not merely on a certain attitude of mind, but rather reflects a particular, worldly disposition of the body. In the midst of his interpretation of the 'sexual' which enters into active, critical dialogue with psychoanalysis, sleep – I argue – turns out, for Merleau-Ponty, to suggest the very image of that 'general form of life' which determines being's embodiment in the world: in other words, perhaps the closest thing to life itself. As he himself puts it, wakefulness and slumber are not 'modalities of consciousness', but rather both sleep and consciousness are expressions of a more basic 'situation' of existence which, however, one would seem to approach more closely in the transit from wakefulness to sleep.

Given the broadly chronological structure of this book, the following chapter turns to a prose text by Paul Celan from the late 1940s, in the process offering what some might see as a 'literary' interlude. Celan's 'dream about the dream' stages a dream-like dialogue or confrontation with the naïvely 'Kleistian' dream of an unnamed 'friend', a crudely 'Kleistian' dream in which meaning and truth is restored to words as the foremost expression of an idyllic return to a prelapsarian world. Celan gives us an *other* dream of this dream, going 'beneath' the paintings of Edgar Jené. It is a surrealist dream-journey that doesn't lead homewards, but instead takes us out to the hithermost side of vision. 'We enter it in our sleep,' writes Celan, 'then we see what remains to be dreamed.'

The next chapter looks at Derrida, Blanchot and Levinas. In Blanchot's *L'Arrêt de mort*, as Derrida suggests, an 'epochal suspension' manifests itself, compulsively pulsating so as to conjure a certain spectrality beyond all consciousness, perception, or ordinary attentiveness. Rereading Blanchot's text, I argue that it is on the borderlines of sleep that the 'arrythmic pulsation' of the *arrêt de mort* happens as impossible event – 'the state of suspension in which it's over – and over again, and you'll never have done with that suspension itself', to quote Derrida once more. While Derrida's 'Living On' makes little of sleep, however, I take this cue to follow a pathway which leads from Blanchot to Levinas. Blanchot's writing exposes the sleep of reason which occurs in the very promise of perfect day, a promise which mutates in the dream he associates with the 'other night', a dream which harbours the irrepressible return of 'time's absence', and which opens on to the very 'outside' which the world – and the self – lacks or wants (as much as 'world' or 'self' seek to overcome this 'outside' as such). Levinas, meanwhile, wants to think irremissible pure existing (*il y a*) in terms of insomnia; in contrast, consciousness seeks to assert itself over the unremitting presence of the 'there is' through its capacity for unconsciousness or sleep. This chapter, then, seeks to attend to the complexities of a certain 'fatality of being' that threatens the 'ego' at the point consciousness's capacity to sleep is confronted by the radical vigilance of insomnia and the deep anonymity of the night (to follow Levinas's *Existence and Existents*).

Chapter Six, starting out as perhaps another 'literary' interlude, turns to the writings of Samuel Beckett, where the possibility of sleep becomes impossibly crossed with the dream of sleep itself, a sleepless dream of sleep, which may indeed lead back to the ever-vigilant anonymity of which Levinas speaks. Beckett's long-acknowledged connection to Descartes, meanwhile, sets the scene for the following chapter, which turns to Derrida's 'Cogito and the History of Madness'. Here, as many will know, the contested interpretation of Descartes's first *Meditation* acquires prominence in Derrida's account of his deep-seated reservations about Foucault's *Madness and Civilization*. Foucault's description of the historical separation of madness from reason is challenged by the fact that, as Derrida sees it, madness is more radically a possibility of reason, to the extent that Descartes's argument has to recognize the possibility of 'thought' being all the while *mad* as it asserts the Cogito (its madness or sanity being inconsequential to the Cogito's certitude). The 'hyperbolical' or 'mad audacity' of the Cogito is therefore prior to the historical separation of what Derrida terms a '*determined* reason' and a '*determined* unreason', and – as a matter of principle – the Cogito remains invulnerable to such a division. Moreover, Derrida suggests that in Foucault's argument about madness, sleep and dreaming are powerfully secondarized in relation to Descartes's project of radicalizing doubt. For Derrida, however, Descartes's allusion to dreams is not to be put to one side in relation to madness. Rather, dreaming for Descartes amounts to 'the hyperbolical exasperation of the hypothesis of madness', as Derrida puts it. Thus, the sleeper or the dreamer is, so Derrida insists, 'madder than the madman'. The chapter gives a full hearing to Foucault's response to Derrida's criticisms, but concludes that, if Derrida is correct in observing that Foucault's interpretation of Descartes foregrounds madness as both doubt's most decisive setting and yet also its most extreme threshold, this very same tension must of necessity upset the demarcation or setting-aside of dreams, which likewise, for Foucault, do not in the end lead into doubt's most intimate interiority. Indeed, since – according to the very trajectory of Foucault's reply to Derrida – the separation of madness from reason depends to a significant extent upon the setting-aside of dreaming within Descartes's discursive practice, I argue that it is the inadequately distinguished figure of sleep which comes back to complicate what is often seen as the absolutely 'confrontational' nature of the Foucault-Derrida dossier.

The book concludes with a chapter on Jean-Luc Nancy's *The Fall of Sleep*, in which, as Nancy remarks, 'sleeping together comes down to sharing an inertia'. For Nancy, sleep's profound unshareability nonetheless provides a telling image of a strange, unworldly commonality: 'an equal world of sleep', as he would have it. As if to confirm the neglected significance of sleep in the 'text' of philosophy, this final chapter traces the frequently unacknowledged philosophical resources of Nancy's book, and wonders about its critical practice as much as the quality of its argument. Sleep for Nancy implies total repose in a fathomless indeterminacy as much as a radically equal 'sharing' beyond any allotted share. It amounts to an overpowering 'fall' in which the constitutive work of difference seems to realize itself in rapturous implosion, as alterity is swept into the abyss of self-abandonment. (I would argue that this 'sweeping away' never quite happens in any of the other authors who feature in *The Poetics of Sleep*, even if it often seems promised or threatened.) If alterity seems to relinquish its own force in Nancy's book, the chapter ends by returning to Derrida, this time his essay 'Violence and Metaphysics', in order to ask about the very possibility of an 'other' beyond the irrecuperable play of *différance* (as, precisely, differentiation's own excess or 'other'). I conclude that the question of the other *drifts* in Nancy's book, and that this 'drift' describes not only the sleep that Nancy wants to write about, but also the manner of Nancy's engagement with a philosophical tradition that remains somewhat inconspicuous throughout his book .

Poiesis of sleep

As is so often the case, the title, *The Poetics of Sleep*, is not mine at all, but instead came from somewhere else. To be more precise, it came from Martin McQuillan, who – as is so often the case – seemed to pull it from nowhere. And it sounded good. Without further thought or reflection, it just sounded like a way to describe what I wanted to do, what I wanted to write. And so I thank him for it, if only according to the multiple tonalities such a phrase acquires.

My first inkling, as McQuillan's title came to dawn on me, was that such a title would neither reduce the subject-matter, nor the task itself, to a more simple expression of disciplinary activity, nor thereby to an exercise of scholarly virtue. Thus, while it was always clear that the book would be concerned with a number of texts one might indeed describe as 'philosophical' (the subheading, of course, firmly indicates a certain philosophical tradition and trajectory), the title McQuillan so audaciously proposed, with his usual intuitive brilliance, stood to one side of that other possibility – *The Philosophy of Sleep* – without, for all that, indicating instead a simple 'literary' turn, at any rate in the sense that a *poetics* of sleep need not imply merely the 'poetry', poeticality or poeticization of sleep (or, therefore, a prettified literary survey in the offing, a somewhat smug 'literary' supplementation or ornamentation of 'the philosophy of sleep', or, for that matter, 'the science of sleep' or 'the politics of sleep', and so on – other possible titles I could no more write under). For, surely, it would be clear to all that the term 'poetics' – as much as standing to one side of it – in fact also leads back to philosophy, perhaps even somewhere close to the origins of philosophy. Or, put differently again, it is doubtless found *on the way* to philosophy, in the sense that for Aristotle the human interest in knowledge leads from *techne* in its different manifestations to philosophy, as arguably a higher yet by no means entirely distinct pursuit. The term 'poetics', we might even say, is to be found at a certain crossroads, between philosophy and literature perhaps, perhaps on the way to somewhere else, somewhere that might yet turn out to be less than remote from either of them.

I mention *techne* here, of course, since in the Greek family of terms to which poetry and poetics belong, *poiesis* is a form of making. I want to say some things about *poiesis* here, therefore, and without delay I want also to acknowledge my indebtedness to another colleague and friend, William Watkin, particularly his book *The Literary Agamben*, which includes some very fine passages on the subject, upon which I draw in the remaining part of this introduction.[15] (Watkin's abiding interest in 'poetic thinking'[16] – to be construed neither simply in terms of 'thinking about poetry', nor just in terms of producing 'thoughtful', 'poetic' texts – itself opens on to a certain trend in post-deconstructive writing, to which my own book may perhaps be considered to contribute in some small way.) In the simplest sense, *poiesis* means 'production'. As Plato famously puts it in the *Symposium*, 'any cause that brings into existence something that was not there before is poiesis'[17] – although we should be careful not to reduce this formulation to that idea of creation which involves an inspired artistic 'will' or masterful genius. For *poiesis* here refers to the fact of a certain process underway, and not merely to the *doing* of an individual (which may nevertheless constitute one form *poiesis* might take, perhaps). Indeed, Aristotle's well-known distinction between *poiesis* and *praxis* establishes itself on the strength of a certain demarcation between production and action, whereby the former term – *poiesis* – describes forms of behaviour aimed at an external end (for example building, the end of which is dwellings or other constructions), in contrast to the latter – *praxis* – which describes acts which take shape as an expression of the will and, more particularly, constitute themselves in terms of the exercise of virtue. Action (*praxis*) in contrast to production (*poiesis*) is to be chosen for its own sake, not simply in the interests of some outcome beyond the specific act that is undertaken. Action, properly speaking, is not a means to an end, but is instead chosen as a matter of prudence, (as) an end in itself. Prudence, virtue, therefore find expression in acts which eschew undue concern for production as, supposedly, a mere means.[18]

As a process (*kinesis*) devoted to an external end or purpose, then, the production involved in *poiesis* is distinct from action construed in terms of acts of virtue which, of necessity or by definition, must be undertaken for their intrinsic value, ethically or morally let's say. *Poiesis*, for Aristotle, is thus characteristic of crafts, and as a form of making is allied with, although it is not simply identical to, *techne*: aside from the fact that the latter conjures a certain notion of technical skill to which *poiesis* is not limited,[19] *techne* for Aristotle is a productive activity that continues to be informed by a sense of its own rationale. However, the knowledge involved in production, making, or craft is not the same as that involved in virtue, notably since the former would seem to include an unreflective dimension (or, rather, it may include something that goes beyond reflection, which remains recalcitrant to reflection or analysis as such). In the *Poetics*, Aristotle is indifferent to the question of whether poets – involved as they are in a certain type of production – have any reflective understanding of their craft. Like other artisans, poets need not understand what it is they are doing, and may be good at it by chance, because of raw talent or instinct, or through simple trial and error. Indeed, the capacity to perceive or convey similarities – so important to poetry as a form of mimesis – is for Aristotle a natural ability that remains essentially unteachable. In *poiesis*, then, everything is a matter of the disposition of materials, whose selection does not necessarily come down to the expression of a will, one that might serve as the determining origin of the creation, or one that might exploit the production as the medium of some 'higher' form of self-reflection.

While *poiesis* as a form of production is not reducible to poetry in the simple sense, nonetheless Aristotle's understanding of the latter is in certain respects illuminating for our understanding of *poiesis* more generally. For Aristotle, poetry is first of all a form of mimesis, although this does not mean poetry is to be understood or evaluated in terms of the production of simple copies or facsimiles of its 'objects', far from it. Poetry as mimesis may produce telling correspondences which need not relate directly either to the content or structure of any given reality. Indeed, *poiesis* more broadly need not necessarily produce 'objects' at all, but merely, if one reads Plato carefully, 'something that was not there before' – a new 'truth' or insight, for instance. Thus, Heidegger defines *poiesis* as that which brings forth into 'uncon-cealment' presences that need not be understood simply in terms of their status as 'objects' (artworks, let's say), but instead as particular combinations of material, form, and purpose which result from the process of making, of which the artistry of the maker may be just one component. As such, *poiesis* unveils or 'makes' truth, or rather it gives rise to a 'mode of truth as unveiling', as Agamben puts it,[20] that is in a certain way embodied by, but is nonetheless not simply identical to, the 'object', relating as it does more to the process of making, the experience of production, than simply to its 'result' (a process or experience which must not, however, be reduced to merely another under-standing of *praxis* or practical action). However, coming back to poetry more specifically, its defining connection to mimesis – or to the mere production of 'similarity' or correspondence – means it retains a constitutive element which resists interpretation based on the discernment or disclosure of *meaning*. Indeed, as Watkin suggests during his discussion of the importance of *poiesis* for the reading of Agamben's work, Aristotle's understanding of poetry as mimesis informs an entire tradition of thought interested in linguistic forms that put in question the idea of the primacy of the conceptual function of language, normally associated with prose.

Poiesis, then, names the production or coming forth of something – not necessarily something as tangible as an 'object', indeed something that essentially remains irreducible to objecthood or objectivity – according to a process which operates at once *beyond* and *below* the level of the will. Something that may well involve the 'will' (volition, agency, rational self-consciousness, autonomous being, the 'active' waking mind, etc.) in its *kinesis*, but only as a component feature – and thus as something 'other' than itself, or 'other' than it would wish to be. (The unconscious may be one name for what we are describing here, although as we shall see, the theory of the unconscious may be as susceptible to what we are seeking to describe as any other form of thought.) Put differently, *poiesis* is at once the doing and undoing of 'man' in the 'world'.[21] And, for Aristotle, *poiesis* is never natural, since natural acts of creation precisely lack the supplementarity of human 'production' (though, in itself, this is both more and less than 'human'); at any rate, the *kinesis* or process that *poiesis* entails is different from the natural act which contains within itself its own *arche*, the origin and principle by which it comes about.

Not quite natural, both beyond and below the level of the will it nevertheless engages, always in excess of thinking or reflection, never reducible to a tangible object, yet ever establishing its rhythms (its arrhythmicality, too) in the space and time of the world,[22] *poiesis* moves among us, between us, makes and unmakes us in all our doings. 'Poeisis makes an outline or contour for being', as Watkin observes (p. 83) – and perhaps productively unworks it, as well. I hope readers of *The Poetics of Sleep* may sense that there might be no better term to couple – or correspond – with sleep than *poiesis*. I hope, too, that *poiesis* may provide an apt term for the 'production' that is this book, as much as it shares a certain affinity with the subject-matter.

1

Philosophy's Limits

Aristotle and the metaphysics of sleep

For Aristotle, sleep and waking are apparently opposite yet fundamentally related phenomena which appertain to a distinct part of the animal, including most especially the human animal. Aristotle understands this special organ in terms of the faculty of 'sense-perception' (as the standard English translation would have it).[1] Thus he argues that, since plant life is incapable of 'sense-perception', plants can neither sleep nor wake. (This is something that, much later on, Bergson among others will re-address.[2]) Aristotle reflects on the fact that sleep appears contrary to, and yet is defined in its relationship with, waking life, in the sense that, if it is indeed construed as the privation of wakefulness (just as sickness is thought to be the privation of health, weakness the privation of strength, and so on), then its definition would nevertheless seem to come from that in relation to which it differs. Indeed, the criterion by which we recognize that a person is awake is identical, observes Aristotle, to the criterion which allows us to perceive the sleeper as asleep: this criterion is that of 'sense-perception' (i.e. it might be said that wakefulness consists in the exercise of such 'sense-perception', which evidently differs in sleep so as to characterize it in relation to wakefulness). In other words, in a move that is absolutely crucial within Aristotle's argument and indeed the philosophical legacy it bequeaths, 'sense-perception' does not just apply to one side of the binary opposition between waking and sleep, but instead organizes both terms. Now, we should be careful in our understanding of what this may mean. As Derrida points out, Heidegger insists that Aristotle connects sleep with neither consciousness nor unconsciousness in the modern sense, but instead says that sleep entails a particular way that *aisthēsis*, as a form of awareness that is not the same thing as pure thought or intellection, is 'bound'. While this would seem to hand down to phenomenology, for instance, the task of a certain rethinking of 'consciousness' (something similar might be said of Bergson, too), it is nevertheless true that the historical reception and translation of Aristotle has had its part to play in the history of a metaphysics that ties sense-perception to (the problem of) consciousness in particular ways.

While sleep may be construed as the privation of wakefulness, Aristotle observes that all animals possessed of sense-perception are incapable of unstinting wakefulness without recourse to sleep. (Equally, there is no animal of this kind who sleeps without ever awakening, precisely since the 'sense-perception' that permits us to 'know' sleep would seem to demand wakefulness as its more 'proper' medium or activity – its very 'goal' (p. 724).) Thus sleep is not merely the privation of wakefulness, but also its necessary supplement. Indeed, during a partly unresolved discussion about whether some types of hard-eyed creatures actually sleep, Aristotle suggests that sleep is, in a certain sense, the very sign by which we recognize the facility of 'sense-perception' in particular life-forms, since in terms of his own argument the inability to sleep indicates precisely the absence of 'sense-perception'. Sleep, then, is inelimi-nable in relation to the function of 'sense-perception' itself. Just as the eyes are weakened by excessively lengthy bouts of looking, or the hand by dint of overly prolonged labour, so the special organ of what we are calling sense-perception requires its own interruption in order to function effectively. This bout of remission, which may be a temporary period of inhibition but also a certain type of transformation, is therefore to be considered restorative.

While sleep may be associated with a certain drifting away of 'sense-perception', Aristotle insists that it requires more specific definition if it is to be delineated in relation to, say, swooning or asphyxia. What characterizes sleep, suggests Aristotle, is that while other forms of sense-deprivation occur in a more extrinsic way, through a chance cause or via some impact on a less fundamental organ of sense (for instance, pressure applied to the blood vessels in the neck), sleep is the seeming privation of 'sense-perception' that, nonetheless, 'sense-perception' gives itself. Sleep, as the English trans-lation of Aristotle has it, finds its 'seat in the primary organ with which one perceives objects in general' (p. 724). Thus, at a more fundamental level, what we are calling sense-perception does not so much lose its power when giving itself over to sleep (the interplay that, as we shall see, Aristotle detects between 'sense-perception' and movement is important here, since the sleeper's ability to move is a sign of the continued activity of the 'primary organ of sense' (p. 725)), and this is why the possibility of sensory perception is not withdrawn absolutely during slumber, instead leaving its impression in dreams.[3]

To explain further why the animal possessed of 'sense-perception' gives itself sleep, Aristotle notes, in particular, that the nutrient part of the animal does its work more efficiently during slumber.[4] Sleep is not simply co-extensive with the total incapacitation of the perceptive faculty, but arises in its specific form (as distinct from fainting or asphyxiation, say) in order to assist the 'evaporation' or 'exhalation attendant upon the process of nutrition' (p. 725). From an early point in his discussion, Aristotle wants to argue that the exercise of 'sense-perception' does not belong exclusively either to the body or the soul: it is instead a movement of the soul through the body. (Once more, Aristotelian thought here bequeaths a certain legacy to the work of, say, Bergson or Merleau-Ponty, as we shall see.) Indeed, Aristotle contends that 'sense-perception' originates in the part of the body which governs movement (including, presumably, this movement of the soul), which for him is the heart. Here, the movement of breathing finds its origin, as does the process of 'cooling' allied to the conservation of heat in the body. But in relation to the nutrient part, digestible matter is, according to Aristotle, taken through a process of movement which drives it upwards, since it must be 'evaporated' (heat, he observes, naturally tends to move in this direction); it then travels back down as it cools, where it tends to re-form as a mass. For Aristotle, this offers a clue as to why bouts of drowsiness are particularly likely to happen after meals (the mass of food 'weighs a person down and causes him to nod, but when it has actually sunk downwards, and by its return has repulsed the hot, sleep comes on' (p. 726)). The same sort of logic is used to explain other conditions, for instance weariness, lethargy, ill-health, and the need for sleep in the young:

> It also follows certain forms of fatigue; for fatigue operates as a solvent, and the dissolved matter acts, if not cold, like food prior to digestion. Moreover, some kinds of illness have this same effect; those arising from moist and hot secretions, as happens with fever-patients and in cases of lethargy. Extreme youth

also has this effect; infants, for example, sleep a great deal, because of the food
being all borne upwards – a mark whereof appears in the disproportionately
large size of the upper parts compared with the lower during infancy, which is
due to the fact that growth predominates in the direction of the former. (p. 726)

For Aristotle, the relatively higher occurrence of epilepsy in the young is also
due to this same upward movement that characterizes their growth and development. Indeed, from the standpoint of this reasoning, Aristotle goes so far
as to liken epilepsy to sleep as a similar kind of seizure: 'For when the spirit
moves upwards in a volume, on its return downwards it distends the veins,
and forcibly compresses the passage through which respiration is effected'
(p. 726). This reasoning concerning the effects of an over-stimulated process
or movement of 'evaporation' or 'exhalation' also explains 'why wines are not
good for infants' (p. 726), and why individuals with large heads (including,
says Aristotle, dwarfs) are prone to excessive sleep!

In sum then, Aristotle states:

> ... sleep is a sort of concentration, or natural recoil, of the hot matter inwards,
> due to the cause above mentioned. Hence restless movement is a marked feature
> in the case of a person when drowsy. But where it begins to fail, he grows cool,
> and owing to this cooling process his eye-lids droop. ... sleep comes on when
> the corporeal element is conveyed upwards by the hot, along the veins, to the
> head. But when that which has been thus carried up can no longer ascend, but
> is too great in quantity it forces the hot back again and flows downwards. Hence
> it is that men sink down when the heat which tends to keep them erect (man
> alone, among animals, being naturally erect) is withdrawn; and this, when it
> befalls them, causes unconsciousness, and afterwards imagination. (p. 727)

Naturally enough, the sleeper awakens once the process of 'digestion' is
completed; that is, when the biological processes as understood by Aristotle
have run their course. This is another absolutely key moment for an entire
history of thinking about sleep's relation to what we have come to call
'consciousness' – and by extension consciousness's relationship to its 'other',
or to its own limits. According to one reading, Aristotle might be taken to
conclude that sleep is largely a physiological response to the natural demands
or workings of the body. According to another, which may not be entirely
opposed to the first (as we shall see throughout this book), sleep is a condition
or function of the organ of 'sense-perception' that is, in an important respect,

the sign of the soul moving through the body. (A further interpretation, one we'll come to, is of the Heideggerian type; while, as we shall also see, a whole host of approaches to the problem of 'consciousness' within the philosophical tradition may be aligned to the problem of reading such passages as we are citing here.) Aristotle writes:

> We have now stated the cause of sleeping, viz., that it consists in the recoil by the corporeal element, borne upwards by the connatural heat, in a mass upon the primary sense-organ; we have also stated what sleep is, having shown that it is a seizure of the primary sense-organ, rendering it unable to actualize its powers; arising of necessity (for it is impossible for an animal to exist if the conditions which render it an animal be not fulfilled), i.e. for the sake of its conservation; since remission of movement tends to the conservation of animals. (p. 728)

This 'seizure' of the primary sense-organ is, let us not forget, a seizure that is also a seizure *of* itself (double genitive). From the perspective of a certain reading of Aristotle, then, sleep emerges as a corporeal solution to the problem of how 'sense-perception' might perpetuate itself, indeed nourish itself, giving to itself an interval of rest and rejuvenation in the interests of its own conservation, without ever relinquishing its seat of power. On this view, sleep might amount to little more than the material substrate and technical prop of the 'sense-perception' that comes to dominate it. Here, 'sense-perception' would give sleep – upon which it depends, conceptually and practically speaking – no other meaning than its own. Thus, by way of a certain – 'philosophical', let's call it – reading or reasoning, 'sense-perception' would be imagined as having the ability to appropriate the 'other' of itself; an 'other' which the very process or necessity of philosophical thought suggests may nevertheless be a dangerous supplement of sorts. Here we find replayed the very deconstructibility of those conceptual terms and pairings which, Derrida has argued, tower over Western thought and culture only at the expense of a certain remainder or supplement that they could never entirely colonize, contain or exclude. (For just this reason, it is perhaps odd that Derrida paid scant attention to the question of sleep in philosophy, as this book will suggest.) Needless to say, the reception of Aristotelian thought over two millenia is replete with assumptions that are far from difficult to identify. For instance, the idea that bodily movement of any kind may be associated with the persistence of 'sense' continues to haunt and horrify the popular imagination. Indeed, at the very limits of life, it continues to inform certain resistances to contemporary medical expertise and practice. For the post-Romantic and post-Freudian imagination, meanwhile, the dream is arguably of special interest precisely since it continues to fascinate as an expression of what might be called sense-perception, at least in a more general sense, whether or not we view dreaming as a function of the perceptual mind, a delusion or distortion of its faculties, or a form of resistance to the power of consciousness (in each of these alternatives, in other words, the dream intrigues us precisely in its *relation* to waking 'sense'). But – given the decon-structibility of a host of inter-related pairs of concepts that have imposed themselves within the Western tradition – what, may we ask, remains of sleep in the philosophical archive (as an archive still to come)? What happens, for instance, at those moments where it is isolated, subordinated and sidelined as a matter of largely physiological interest, while at the same time being recouped in the process of metaphysical thought re-tooling itself? What will sleep have become, in the 'text' of Western metaphysics? How does it get embroiled in the gaps, tensions and contradictions which in fact make such a 'text' possible? If Aristotle's undoubtedly complex – and indeed contestable – attitude to sleep and waking somewhat dictates the philosophical terrain from which subsequent writings about sleep and dreaming continue to emerge, what is the specificity of each in relation to this inheritance? Which among them are the more powerfully deciphering and, indeed, transformative?

Re-reading Aristotle, or, animal sleep

Here, before continuing on our journey through the 'text' of philosophy, it may be useful to re-open the question of the 'animal' and of 'man' that is suggested by Aristotle's treatise on sleep, in order (as we've already suggested) to multiply its possible readings. In Derrida's *The Animal That Therefore I Am*,[5] the question of sleep and dreaming for what is called 'man' and what is called 'animal' becomes important on more than one occasion. For Derrida, of course, the 'animal' question has a structuring importance throughout the entire 'text' of philosophy: in particular, the term 'animal' has been used right across philosophical history to found and maintain a classical opposition through which the concept of the 'human' may be proposed in binary terms. Thus, what might be presumed to be 'proper' to the human – including, in Derrida's own list, language, speech, reason, the experience or possibility of death *as such*, the possibility of mourning, the existence of culture, institutions, or technics, the possibility of the gift, of laughter, tears, lying, respect, and so forth – is frequently brought to the fore through the negative determination of the 'animal' as binary opposite. From Aristotle to Heidegger, from Descartes to Kant, Levinas and Lacan, Derrida suggests, there has been a tendency to deny the animal the *logos*. (In one sense, we might say, the *logos* and thus philosophy in its classical sense is founded upon the 'animal' as oppositional 'other'; that is, as at once the object of appropriation and yet also a projection of philosophy's or indeed humanity's own – albeit enabling – limitations.) Furthermore, the homogenizing concept and category of the 'animal' offers violence both to the sheer diversity of animal life and to the irreducibly complex and always deconstructible relation of the 'animal' to the 'human'.

Here, Derrida explores the question of dreaming in certain animals, which he argues is somewhat analogous to other questions which seek to distinguish the animal from the human, for instance 'does the animal think?', 'does the animal have a language?', etc. With some recourse to available scientific and zoological knowledge, Derrida speculates that dreaming is sufficiently differentiated among various types of animal that one should in fact speak of '(the) animals' rather than the animal *as such*, 'renouncing any horizon of unification of the concept of the animal' and indeed calling into question the conceptual pairing/opposition of animal – man. Indeed, he suggests that certain key differences in dreaming may well connect some 'animals' to 'man' just as much as they might separate some 'animals' from each other.

Derrida therefore challenges the grounds of the opposition between the 'human' and the 'animal'. In the last part of the book, for example, during an improvised speech on Heidegger and the animal, he points up the contradictions which run through Heideggerian thought on this very subject. For at one moment, in comparison to *Dasein*, the animal is excluded from 'being-towards-death', and as such does not properly die. And yet, at another time, the animal is accorded the character of a living being, in contrast to the inanimate or 'worldless' stone, suggesting the very possibility of dying which is common to 'man'. Derrida thereby suggests at once the limits and exemplarity of the

Heideggerian 'text' on the animal. For, here, the animal both *does* and *does not* have the 'as such' which founds the possibility of the *logos*, and indeed this difference-beyond-opposition calls for new forms of thinking – ethical as much as philosophical – which cannot be based simply on the 'as such' and its absence or deprivation. Thus, Derrida suggests the need for a rigorous and transforming reinvestigation, rather than a simple defence, of 'human rights' and 'animal rights' – something which calls for a more fundamental questioning of what is meant by 'life', both within and beyond philosophical thought.

To come back to the question of sleep, however, the section of *The Animal That Therefore I Am* which concerns Heidegger is particularly interesting (not least, since it doesn't just aim at the deconstructibility of Heideggerian thought, but also implicitly foregrounds such thought as another reading of 'metaphysics' that goes via Aristotle). Here, we find Derrida reminding us that in *Being and Time* what is connected to the question of the modalities of being is the idea not just of employing something that is ready-to-hand, but – with 'more radical reach', as Derrida puts it – of 'letting what is asleep become wakeful' (p. 147). The significance acquired by awakening[6] in this Heideggerian discourse therefore implies the (philosophical) importance of the question of sleep, and, as Derrida is quick to point out, Heidegger insists that the relationship between waking and sleeping cannot be reduced or collapsed into a distinction between consciousness and unconsciousness. 'What he calls waking is not consciousness; what he calls sleeping is not the unconscious', Derrida thus says of Heidegger (p.147). In turn, Derrida shows that this way of thinking – whereby awakening is linked to a certain 'attunement' which cannot be reduced to the passage from unconsciousness to consciousness – seeks to 'define the essence of the human otherwise than through consciousness, otherwise than through the reason that might be attributed to a certain animal' (p. 148); otherwise, that is, than through a distinction between 'mind' and matter which produces a certain discourse of 'man' and of the 'animal'. From this, Derrida observes that Heidegger is as compelled as Freud was to confront 'the question of what happens when an animal sleeps' (p. 148). In fact, for Derrida this issue runs right across the philosophical heritage that he wants to address. Heidegger has trouble answering the question of whether a plant sleeps (although he seems to have no difficulty dealing with this matter in regard to the stone), making the uncertainty of his response on the issue equivalent to that which follows from the question of whether the plant is ever in any sense 'awake'.[7] Furthermore, while we 'know' that the animal sleeps, says Heidegger, we cannot be sure of the nature of this sleep in regard to the sleep of 'man', and, to go further, we do not yet know what we really mean by sleep *in general*. Since Heidegger wants to put the question of sleep and awakening (itself construed as a question concerning the very structure of being) in a way that resists or transforms a certain metaphysics of consciousness, he seeks another path, by which the question of sleep is further complicated. Here, Derrida turns to some remarks by Heidegger on Aristotle. In *Being and Time*, Heidegger insists that Aristotle links sleep with neither consciousness nor unconsciousness (in the sense these terms have developed since his own time). Instead, for Heidegger, Aristotle thinks of sleep as basically a '*desmos*', that is, a 'being bound' or a certain way that *aisthēsis* undergoes binding (*aisthēsis* refers to a form of perception or sensation, in short an awareness, that differs from intellection or pure thought). As we shall see, such a conception of sleep may well return in phenomenological discourse, particularly that of Merleau-Ponty. However, Derrida speculates from this that Heidegger would understand the relation of the 'human' and of the 'animal' to sleep in terms of a different manner of 'being bound', rather than in terms of an opposition between consciousness and unconsciousness which conventionally divides 'man' from all others more decisively. Thus Heidegger speaks of what is 'bound' as not only our 'perception' but also 'our essence', through which 'it cannot take in other beings which it itself is not'.[8] Hence, as Derrida notes, 'the animal is too well bound', yet this very same binding does not decisively separate 'man' from 'animal' since, on Heidegger's reading of Aristotle, man's 'essence' also involves a question of what is 'bound'. In this passage from *Being and Time*, then, the question of sleep opens up a 'broad perspective which has by no means been grasped in its metaphysical intent', as Heidegger puts it; nevertheless, interestingly and perhaps tellingly, for 'fundamental metaphysical reasons' he foregoes the question of sleep (in its own right?) in favour of taking another pathway concerning the problem of 'what it means to awaken an attunement'. But still, it is important to note here that Heidegger attempts another reading of Aristotle than the one which imputes to his discourse the origins of a modern notion of consciousness which came to dominate thought – and to exercise it – in the centuries to come.

Kant: Sleep from a pragmatic point of view

In philosophy (though doubtless beyond philosophy, too), there is a certain tradition of viewing sleep as the dutiful prop and productive supplement of daytime tasks and responsibilities, or, to go further, a rational instrument of rational life. As we have said, a certain reading of Aristotle participates in this tendency. To travel forward in time several millennia from Aristotle's day, in *Anthropology from a pragmatic point of view*,[9] for instance, Kant defines sleep as 'a condition in which a healthy human being is unable to become conscious of representations through the external senses'. It is, thus, 'a relaxation, which is nevertheless at the same time a gathering of power for renewed external sensations' (p. 276). In a subsequently crossed-out footnote to this very same passage, Kant speculates that excessive and thus non-instrumental sleep may result in early death, in rather the same way that gluttony, for 'the Mohammedan', risks using up a lifetime's proportion of food too soon. Sleep is thus to be restricted to its proper place, quantity and time, in order that it effectively serve the interests of the day. While Kant has no problem in describing dreaming during sleep as evidence of a 'healthy condition', he is quick to add that 'if it happens while the human being is awake, it reveals a diseased condition' – diseased, presumably, because wakeful dreaming uncomfortably disturbs the clear boundary that grants sleep its primary function, namely 'the recovery of powers expended while awake' (p. 285). (To the extent that sleep and dreaming are the rational instrument of rational life, Kant is unable to propose, within the field of '*pragmatic* anthropology', the 'rules of *conduct*' of somnambulism, since such rules – the very rules which allow us to judge sleeping from a pragmatic point of view – would only be valid for the wholly supine, deep-dreaming slumberer or the clear-eyed, undreaming man of the day.[10] Thus, the 'Greek emperor who condemned a human being to death when he explained to his friends that in his dream he had killed the emperor' acts, Kant insists, in a way that is 'both contrary to experience and cruel', mistaking as he does the clear distinction between sleep and wakefulness which permits 'conduct' to be judged appropriately).

Having stated that night-time dreaming is indeed healthy, Kant adds that dreams keep life 'active' during sleep and thus bar the passage to total sleep, or in other words to an unagitated, unanimated slumber which would in fact signal death itself. This 'functional' attitude to dreaming is, of course, merely the obverse of what we might loosely term the post-Romantic, post-Freudian (and, to some extent, neuro-scientific) mindset, one which largely thinks of the dream as either a processing-device for the remnants of waking thought or unresolved psychic material, or perhaps more darkly as a night-time terror that engages the psyche in something like a fight for survival, thus providing the means for the 'mind' to re-establish its powers in view of the onset of coming day (even if only in terms of its imaginative capabilities, if not its analytical powers). Indeed, Kant himself tells a personal anecdote which illustrates the 'beneficial effect of dreaming during a so-called *nightmare*' (p. 298). He relates a childhood dream of drowning which he feels sure quickened his failing breathing while asleep, waking him temporarily, and thus saving his life.

Kant's notion of the workings of the sleeper's dream resonates somewhat with Herschel Farbman's recent contention that the dream constitutes 'the internal boundary' that makes sleep possible – while also making full sleep quite impossible.[11] In his survey of certain key twentieth-century writers and thinkers, including Freud, Blanchot, Joyce and Beckett, Farbman shows how the dream can be thought of in this way. Since total sleep (complete and thus perpetual repose) would be tantamount to death, as Kant himself suggests, it would bring sleep to an irrevocable end. Dreaming is thus, as Farbman puts it, the very difference between sleep and death – and for 'post-Romantic' or 'post-Freudian' thought it is therefore, perhaps, the essential threshold between the two. Furthermore, the twentieth century, 'post-Freud', has conceived of sleep and dreaming in a way that often merely rethinks the implications of Kant's anecdote on a grand scale, arguing not so much that dreaming defends the otherwise inattentive sleeper against the actual onset of death, but – as the reverse side of this argument – that dreams incorporate and negotiate psychic disturbances inherited from the day so that, rather than the sleeper being awoken by such anxieties, sleep is prolonged for an amount of time that is conducive to the very 'rest' that, from one point of view, remains essential for the prolongation of life. (Later on, we will look in more detail at the connection of these ideas to Freudian thought.) In other words, within this broad viewpoint, 'life' enters into dreams – albeit in a number of ways, and with a number of different results – primarily in order to preserve or nurture 'life' itself. The rest that sleep may give us – which, Freud argues, is as much guarded as threatened by dreams[12] – may of course be imagined simply in terms of physical repose, but is also often thought about in terms of a certain degree of psychological recuperation or benefit – even if the dreams experienced during sleep seem unremittingly disturbing.[13] (As we saw in the introduction, such thinking provokes significant discussion within contemporary sleep research and science.) However, to the extent that the mind's rest, as well as the body's, may be at stake in sleep, for Freud any beneficial dimension of sleeping frequently comes at the price of the persistence of anxiety (although Freud himself is relatively immune, as a long-term sound sleeper, at any rate if *The Intepretation of Dreams* is to be believed[14]). In Farbman's description of *The Interpretation of Dreams* the dream is portrayed as an attempt 'to maintain the sleep that is the condition of its own production' while at the same time defending against radical separation and death precisely by including day-time matter, thus retaining 'open connections to the world against the subject's wish to withdraw completely into itself' (pp. 42–3).[15] As Farbman would have it, then, dreaming for Freud 'maintains the thread of experience over the radical gap in experience ... that sleep represents' (p. 45), even if the process through which such a 'thread' is maintained originates in the dream-work as radically prior or excessive in relation to the subject of just such a 'relation'.[16] While far from becoming its out-and-out enemy, the dream thus resists sleep in its fullest sense, maintaining the connection to day-time life albeit by means of a 'work' which cannot simply be reincorporated or reappropriated by the day (or, in other words, by the rational subject). For modern thought, one might say, the dream impedes as much as it facilitates the seemingly intrinsic (yet, equally, impossible) double momentum that orients sleep towards the day, on the one hand, while driving it towards death, on the other.

The profound complications – and the production of anxiety – that this situation entails are, for sure, not yet fully worked out in Kant's text. 'Dreaming', Kant concludes, is merely 'a wise arrangement of nature for exciting the power of life through affects related to involuntary and invented events, while bodily movements based on choice, namely muscular movements, are in the meantime suspended' (p. 285). Indeed, Kant implies that individuals forget a large proportion of their dreams as precisely an extension of this 'wise arrangement of nature'; that is to say, dreams are by and large forgotten in order to discourage the delusion of an 'actual' shadowy existence in an alternative night-time universe, or, put differently, to rebut the idea of an otherworldly somnambulism that genuinely takes place during sleep. Sleep and dreaming are, then, to be thought of as principally rational tools of non-deadly rest; albeit tools which, through misuse, or misadventure outside the rational field, nonetheless make possible certain hazards: delusion, sleep-walking, irrational conduct, a propensity to excessive sleep, and thus perhaps premature death. (Hazards which are in one sense fated by the conceptual restriction of sleep to its own functionality.)

Hegel: Sleep and being-for-self

In his *Philosophy of Mind*,[17] meanwhile, Hegel's understanding of dreams resonates with Bergson's idea, emerging almost a century later, that dreaming is not so much the result of the unconscious mind working in a complex and dissonant relation to consciousness, as it is simply the product of 'the entire mental life minus the effort of concentration'. (We will come back to Bergson in the next chapter, notably in relation to Freud.) For Bergson, what we experience in dreams occurs through a particular combination of sensation and memory. Although it happens in a different way, this same interplay also shapes our day-time awareness, he argues. Thus, dreaming and wakefulness are not merely opposed states. Instead, they are just different forms of experience or perception, whereby a certain type of 'tension' that characterizes the processing of sensation in waking life (a processing continually subjected to probabilistic interpretations of experience) is replaced by 'extension' (that is to say, more freely associative thoughts or images in dreams). Put simplistically, during dreaming our memory – having been sparked by sensation – becomes 'unconcentrated', as it were. While we are awake, however, the effort of 'concentration' means that sensation is processed by the memory in a dissimilar manner. For Bergson it is almost as if, from sheer necessity, consciousness works rather precipitately in forming perceptions through the 'tension' or 'concentration' it brings to bear on experience (so that consciousness is, in a sense, less responsive than the dream to the entire field of possibility opened up as sensation puts memory to work). For Hegel, however, the 'wild disorder' (as he puts it) of dreams is to be understood through a differently developed sense of what constitutes the waking mind. In contrast to Bergson's notion of the hyper-alert dream (according to which wakefulness is really a type of restriction of full consciousness), Hegel insists that dreams break up the 'concrete' connections that result from the waking mind operating in its own interests as a 'totality':

> In dreams our attitude is only representational; there our representations are not governed by the categories of the intellect. But mere representation wrests things completely out of their concrete interconnection, individualizes them. Hence in dreams everything drifts apart, criss-crosses in wild disorder, objects lose all necessary, objective, intellectual, rational interconnection and only enter into an entirely superficial, contingent and subjective combination. Thus it happens that we bring something we hear in sleep into an entirely different context from what it has in actuality. One hears, for example, a door slam, believes a shot has been fired, and now pictures a story of robbers ... The occurrence of such false representations in sleep is possible because in this state the mind is not the totality for itself, with which, in waking, it compares all its sensations, intuitions, and representations, in order to ascertain, from the agreement or non-agreement of the individual sensations, intuitions, and representations with its totality, a totality that is for itself, the objectivity or non-objectivity of that content. (p. 67)

Here, then, while the contemplation of dreaming is as crucial to Hegel as it is to Bergson in developing a theory of what consciousness means, Hegel sides with the idea that probabilistic interpretation – rather than just amounting to a tactical restriction in the interests of ongoing survival or the contingencies of 'good sense' – expresses the full being-for-self of the waking 'self'. As a consequence, though dreams are an important instrument in thinking about the waking mind, it becomes possible for Hegel to trivialize them in a way that Bergon's thought will not allow. In other words, dreams do not so much open up the total field of the mind's workings, in contrast to the restricted or 'concentrated' perceptions called for by wakefulness; instead, they are just what happens to perception when the self as a 'totality for itself' loosens its grip:

> Only occasionally does something occur in a dream that has a significant connection with actuality. This is especially so with dreams before midnight; in these the representations can still to some extent be held in an orderly connection with the actuality with which we have occupied ourselves in the daytime. At midnight, as thieves very well know, we sleep soundest; the soul has then withdrawn into itself away from all tension with the external world. After midnight, dreams become even more arbitrary than before. (p. 67)

While it is no doubt possible to view Hegel's calibration of night as a presentiment of the latter-day, scientific study of sleep (which tells us much about dreaming in the early phase of sleep and in later REM sleep), what is more interesting in this passage is the distinction that begins to emerge between the 'soul' as that which becomes 'withdrawn into itself' during sound sleep, and the mind as that which fully intervenes during the day in order to ensure 'being-for-self'. Whizzing forward in time to the near present-day, in *The Fall of Sleep* Jean-Luc Nancy's idea of an undifferentiated sleeping self, a self unmediated by all the demarcations and discriminations of the day-time and thus wholly abandoned to itself – while at the same time, and for precisely the same reasons, losing all distinction *as such* – no doubt echoes Hegel in a certain way (we will return to Nancy in more detail near the end of this book). Indeed, in a rare moment of explicit reference to the philosophical tradition of writing about sleep, Nancy cites Hegel's remark, in this same first section of the *Philosophy of Mind*, that sleep is 'the state where the soul is plunged into its undifferentiated unity – waking, on the other hand, is the state in which the soul has entered into opposition to this simple unity'. Taken alone, however, this quotation suggests (to the untrained eye) that the 'soul' is to be viewed simply as an ideal form, to which wakefulness does a certain violence. But, as the text proceeds, Hegel talks about the soul rather differently. In discussing somnambulance as a type of illness, the general characteristics of which are shared with catalepsy and St Vitus's dance, he suggests that the sleepwalker has fallen prey to a particular dysfunction whereby:

> the merely *soulful* side of the organism, becoming independent of the power of *mental* consciousness, usurps the latter's function and the mind, in losing

> control of the soulful component belonging to it, no longer remains in command
> of itself but itself sinks to the form of the soulful and in this way surrenders the
> objective relation to the actual world essential to the sound mind. (p. 98)

Thus, the withdrawal-into-itself of the 'soul' during sleepwalking – since it comes at the price of excluding 'the power of *mental* consciousness' – far from results in a happy or rapturous unity. On the contrary, the full abandonment of the soul to itself in fact militates against being-for-self, since by foregoing 'the objective relation to the actual world' the self risks not only its sanity but its very integrity as such. Nancy borrows from Hegel, therefore, while at the same time declining to take up certain of the implications of his thought (whether for good reason or not).

Despite the implied menace that lurks deep in the heart of sleep – for the withdrawal into itself of the 'soul' in soundest slumber looks to be both an unavoidable or natural fact and at the same time the very basis for the disorder of somnambulism – Hegel well appreciates that the waking mind needs it. However, Hegel's argument here is philosophical, as it were, rather than simply physiological. He writes:

> Finally we must add that waking, as a natural state, as a natural tension between
> the individual soul and the external world, has a *limit*, a measure, that therefore
> the activity of the waking mind gets tired and so induces sleep which, on its side,
> likewise has a limit and must progress to its opposite. (p. 67)

Precisely because the waking self is defined by limits, for instance the limits it sets on dream-like 'representations' in the interests of being-for-self, it must live by the very law of the limit which determines its character. Wakefulness is, in nature, the limit which not simply divides the 'individual soul' from the 'external world' but which makes possible the very compromise between the two, a compromise that results in the mind's ascendancy. Through its 'natural' relationship to the limit (a limit that it itself *is*), the mind must, naturally, accede to its own limits, the natural expression of which is ... sleep. And since sleep is just this natural expression of the law of limitations, it too must succumb to a natural restriction which ensures daily awakening. In Farbman's book, as we have suggested, the dream is often presented – in terms of post-psychoanalytic thought – as that which insures against full sleep which, in its totality, would be nothing other than death. In Hegel's argument, however, it is not the dream that is required to arrest sleep and thus protect the sleeper from his own impending demise. Instead, sleep is curtailed – naturally – by the law that gives us consciousness, rather than by a darker law that dredges dreams from the unconscious in order to reawaken (a semblance of) consciousness itself. Put differently, the reawakening of the conscious mind does not depend on a supplementary 'other', but occurs instead simply on the basis of the law with which consciousness provides itself. In the process, this argument begins to ward off the troubling idea, emerging several pages on, that the sickness implied by sleepwalking might be traced back to sleep itself (since in both cases Hegel suggests that the soul cuts loose from the controls of the mind in its highly regulated relation to the external world). In this earlier part of the text, then, the trail begins to go cold which suggests that illness or disorder may be due to an inherent imbalance in sleep, and instead Hegel seeks to draw our eye with the idea that sleep is nothing but the true expression of nature, order, proper measure.

From this point onwards, Hegel deliberates the dialectical relation of sleep to waking, in terms of a movement towards a 'concrete unity' that transcends their separate determinations. Such a unity is, however, 'always only striven for', precisely to the extent that what 'comes to *actuality* in the *sentient* soul' remains the product of just this ceaseless or inherent 'alternation' between waking and sleeping. As this line of reasoning proceeds, once more the soul is given a more positive spin in terms of its relationship to being-for-self:

> Thus the *abstract* being-for-self present in awaking obtains its first fulfilment through the determinations which are implicitly contained in the soul's sleeping nature, in the soul's substantial being. Actualized, assured, by this fulfilment, the soul proves to itself its being-for-self, its awokeness: it not merely is for itself, it also posits itself as for itself, as subjectivity, as negativity of its immediate determinations. Thus the soul has first attained its *genuine* individuality. This subjective point of the soul now no longer stands isolated, confronting the immediacy of the soul, but asserts itself in the manifold which is contained, in potentiality, in that immediacy. (p. 68)

It turns out that, now, the being-for-self which had previously been characterized in terms of the necessary precedence of '*mental* consciousness' over an otherwise potentially distended and disordered soul should in fact be understood in terms of a more holistic or symbiotic relationship between the two. For without the substance offered by the soul, mental life produces being-for-self only abstractly or mechanically. Once more, nature shifts back towards the soul – or, rather, in the depths of its sleep we find nature's substance rather than unnatural sickness. What we find in 'the soul's sleeping nature' therefore brings 'mental consciousness' to life, it does nothing less than enliven or awaken it. Thus the soul is far from somnambulant (i.e. operating independently from the power of the waking mind): it is 'awokeness' itself. In the purity or 'fulfilment' of this identity, it no longer threatens but instead encapsulates being-for-self. Once again, Hegel has headed off the implications of his own suggestion that the disorder of somnambulism is not simply an anomaly but a particular expression of that which occurs in sleep. In the process, the soul is no longer 'isolated' in its own immediacy. Instead, it has found a place in the determination of being-for-self which previously had derived from the operations of the 'mental consciousness' alone. Awake, 'assured', it asserts and indeed 'posits' itself as if it were now entirely congruous with mental life. Thus the opposition between 'being-for-self or its subjectivity and its immediacy or its substantial being-in-self' is sublated (pp. 68–9). However, *as* sublation, this does not happen 'in *such* a manner that, in the return of awaking into sleep, its being-for-self makes room for its opposite, that mere being-in-self, but so that its being-for-self preserves itself in the alteration, in the Other, develops and proves itself, and the soul's immediacy is reduced from the form of a state present *alongside* that being-for-self to a determination subsisting only *in* that being-for-self, reduced, consequently, to a *semblance*' (p. 69). Being-for-self does not win out simply by including its opposite *as* opposite or distinct 'other' (what Freud would call incorporation), but does so instead by working on, transforming that seeming opposite so that it becomes precisely the intrinsic element it was always bound to become (what Freud would call introjection). Being-for-self does not just want to dominate by preserving and ruling over the otherness of its other (being-in-self), but rather it seeks a more profound victory by dint of dialectical transcendence of the opposition in a new form or new understanding of being-for-self. Hence, the potential menace of the imbalanced or excessive 'soulfulness' of the sleeping soul – a menace that actualizes itself in sleepwalking – turns out to have been a false or at least temporary problem for Hegelian thought, as being-in-self is re-actualized as an expression-without-remainder of being-for-self.

Nonetheless, the category of the other is not cancelled forthwith, far from it. It has a further job to do in getting us to being-for-self. Hegel writes that, upon awakening:

> we find ourselves initially in an entirely indeterminate distinguishedness from the external world generally. Only when we start to sense does this distinction become a *determinate* distinction. In order, therefore, to attain to full wakefulness and certainty of it, we open our eyes, take hold of ourselves, in a word, examine whether some determinate Other, something determinately distinct from ourselves, is for us. In this examination we no longer relate ourselves to the Other, but *mediately*. Thus for example, *contact* is the mediation between myself and the Other, since though it is different from these two sides of the opposition, yet at the same time it unites them both. (p. 69)

The *mediate* rather than immediate relation to the Other is what gives us the 'concrete' conditions or 'interconnections' which the waking self must decide upon precisely in order to express being-for-self. An unmediated or direct relation to the Other would potentially be as bad for being-for-self as the total abandonment to being-in-self that leads to an uncontrolled 'soulful component' driving the sleeper to somnambulance. Thus, Hegel argues that the soul in fact joins together with itself 'after dividing itself in awaking' (i.e. positing or acknowledging itself *as such* rather than remaining isolated in mere immediacy or being-in-self), precisely by means of 'the mediation of something standing between itself and the Other'. The self joins to itself, that is, by means of 'the sensed content' that stands between (and mediates) myself and the Other. By this means, the self 'reflects itself out of the Other into itself, separates itself from the Other and thereby confirms to itself its being-for-self'. This Hegel calls the 'advance' that the 'soul' makes 'by its transition to sensation'.

In just this selection of privileged texts from within the philosophical corpus, then, the image of sleep traverses an increasingly recognizable – if intensifyingly dense – set of possibilities. These range from sleep as largely a physiological condition and question (thus, somewhat marginal to philosophy) to the idea of sleep as at bottom the expression of a 'self' or 'mind', the instrument and effect of 'sense-perception' or, to go further, 'consciousness'. (Indeed, the emergence of sleep as a philosophical topic frequently becomes most interesting where the inter-implication of these two main possibilities arises; where, as the 'text' of philosophy unfolds, far from continuing to function as the mutually exclusive alternatives or complementary unities they might at first glance seem to be, the 'physiological' and the 'psychic' complexly – and often deconstructibly – intersect one another.) Furthermore, across these examples from ancient and enlightenment philosophy, a strange legacy is bequeathed to thought, whereby, in the very attempt to rationalize sleep in terms of its functional or harmonious relationship to both bodily and waking life, a certain supplement is unleashed – call it somnambulance, or some other name – which, in its more troublesome guises, cannot be excluded, contained or sidelined without difficulty.

Freudian Sleep

Bergson and the mental life of sleep

In response to the equally unsatisfactory alternatives of religious interpretation and scientific neglect, not all forms of thought on the cusp of the
twentieth century chose to highlight the influence of the unconscious on
dreams, and not all thinkers were unwary of its snares. For instance, Bergson,
writing at the turn of the century, argues that the explanation of dreams lies
less in the deeply submerged workings of the unconscious than in the role
played by external stimuli as they continue to impress themselves upon the
sleeper's eye, body, and mind.[1] It is, then, the external world, and not the
inner workings of the unconscious, that is responsible for calling up the
memories played out in dreams. Bergson writes, 'in natural sleep our senses
are by no means closed to external impressions ... it is out of real sensation
that we fabricate the dream' (p. 89), and he goes on to describe the dream as
'a resurrection of the past' (p. 90) only in a very particular (and principally
non-Freudian[2]) sense. For him, the welter of memories – some recognized,
others not – that are unleashed in the sleeper's mind 'rise and spread abroad'
during a 'wild phantasmagoric dance' which sees only some get through
the half-ajar 'door' to which they 'rush' during night-time repose. Among
the multitude of recollections stored in the mind, then, the dreamer recalls
some rather than others on the basis that they somehow connect with the
actual or physical sensations experienced while asleep. Thus, 'among the
phantom memories which aspire to weight themselves with colour, with
sound, in short with materiality, those only succeed which can assimilate
the colour-dust I perceive, the noises within and without that I hear, etc.,
and which, besides, are in harmony with the general affective state which

my organic impressions compose. When this union between memory and sensation is effected, I dream' (p. 93).[3] For Bergson, however, perception is far from 'narrowed' during sleep. (In *The Interpretation of Dreams*, published just two years earlier, Freud himself rails against those that view dreaming as merely the product of a partial consciousness and who thus see it as simply a privative, defective version of the waking state proper.) Rather, for Bergson, perception if anything *widens* 'its field of operation' during slumber.[4] While asleep, perception only 'loses in *tension* what it gains in extension', he writes (p. 89). Bergson argues that a dream is in fact 'elaborated almost in the same way as perception of the real world. The mechanism of this operation is the same in its main lines. For what we see of an object placed before our eyes, what we hear of a sentence pronounced in our ear, is trifling in comparison to what our memory adds to it' (p. 94). Whereas during the waking hours perception functions to process 'real impressions made on the organs of sense' more quickly, by subjecting them to memory and 'logic' in order to filter possibilities and thus arrive at a probabilistic interpretation of experience, the dreaming mind is far less susceptible to this particular kind of processing. This is not to say that the dreamer is merely 'irrational'. On the contrary, since the waking mind hastily discounts alternatives in its quest to rationalize experience, it in fact sets aside key features of rationalist enquiry, preferring memory and crude probability to do the work of interpretation on a day-to-day and indeed moment-by-moment basis. Such an effort, whereby at every turn 'the whole memory', all 'accumulated experience', is suddenly 'compressed' in order that it can 'converge' on and interpret a given sensation or stimulus is of course not acknowledged by the waking self as the process of 'choice' or selection it in fact truly is. Thus in a certain sense, waking perception is more half-asleep than the perception that happens in dreams, even though – *indeed, due to the very fact that* – the sleeper is as Bergson puts it 'detached from life' and thus a figure of disinterestedness itself. But perhaps most significantly, by way of this argument Bergson is able to suggest that the dream is neither a partial and derivative form of consciousness, as many in the late nineteenth century would have insisted, nor a wholly separate realm of perception or experience governed by a deep-seated unconscious. Rather, wakefulness and dreaming simply constitute different or differential reactions to the same interplay, i.e. that which occurs between sensation and memory. Thus the dream is just 'the entire mental life minus the effort of concentration' (p. 100), as Bergson famously puts it. (In 'Sleep, Night', one of the appendices of *The Space of Literature*, Blanchot cites Bergson on precisely this point: 'Bergson said that sleep is distinterestedness. Perhaps sleep is inattention to the world, but this negation of the world conserves us for the world and affirms the world.'[5] Here, Bergson's larger attempt to theorize dreams in a way that resists the main trajectory of certain forms of psychological interpretation while refraining from the intellectually suspect and rather retrogressive explanations of the time seems of less interest to Blanchot than his own desire to cite Bergson rather cursorily in order to condemn day-oriented understandings of sleep and dreaming, even though dream-perception in Bergson in fact links to a form of philosophy which aims to think 'beyond' the subject as origin or telos.[6])

Freud and the interpretation of sleep

In *The Interpretation of Dreams*,[7] meanwhile, Freud – also writing on the cusp of the new century – acknowledges that unresolved psychic remainders left over from the waking day do commonly enter into dreams, and indeed play an important part in them. Nevertheless, on several occasions he wants to insist that they do not provide the primary explanation for dreams. For instance, in the chapter 'On Wish-Fulfilment' found in the last section of the book, Freud speaks of a dream of his that is apparently borne of a 'worry', one 'that had my friend Otto appear with the symptoms of Basedow's disease'. On closer analysis, however, Freud is able to explain this dream in terms of his own, personal 'rage for greatness' (pp. 364–5). Freud therefore suggests that, in this case, day-time residues supply only the 'material for active sensations during sleep', as he puts it, rather than forming the basis for the dream's deeper interpretation:

> I grant that there is an entire group of dreams which are *initiated* mainly, or even exclusively, by the remains of the day... But even so, the worry [which is yet 'stirring from the day'] should still not have produced a dream; the *driving-force* that the dream needed had to be contributed by a wish; it was up to the worry to find a wish for itself that would act as the driving-force of the dream. (p. 365)

Freud explains the persistence in dreams of thought-processes carried over from the day in a number of ways. Such residues may be the result of unsolved problems, unresolved cares, or other striking 'impressions' that have not been adequately dealt with in waking life, due to some chance hindrance, or the lack of psychic capacity, or some other form of suppression. He writes, 'there is no need to underestimate the psychical intensities that these remains of the day introduce into the condition of sleep, especially from the group of unresolved problems'. Nonetheless, just a few lines later, Freud is quick to add that, notwithstanding the significant 'changes of energy charge' introduced into the psychic system generally by the state of sleep, 'there is nothing I know of in the psychology of dreams that bids us assume that sleep is anything but a secondary factor' in bringing about changes in the system of the unconscious (p. 364). The materials carried over into dreaming under the specific circumstances of sleep do not fundamentally create the conditions for the transformation of the unconscious, but instead constitute themselves as merely a 'secondary factor' in any changes it might undergo. In this respect, the impact upon dreaming of psychic residues from the day-time, as they are transformed under the conditions of sleep, is at once admitted and strongly qualified in relation to the fundamental power or structural force of the unconscious. Indeed, a little earlier, Freud tells us that he believes 'the wish left unfulfilled from the day is not strong enough in adults to create a dream': it may 'contribute towards arousing the dream', but the latter would not arise if the dream had no other source where it could get reinforcement. Thus, Freud asserts the principle that '*the conscious wish becomes the initiator of a dream only if it succeeds in awakening an unconscious wish consonant with it*' (p. 362), such that 'wishful impulses arising from conscious waking life' must retain a secondary position with regard to the question of dream formation, taking a backseat in relation to analytic enquiry into the unconscious itself.

For Freud, then, the dream is not what it is for Bergson. For Bergson, dreaming is just the ongoing product of a particular interaction between sensation and memory forged during sleep, as the whole mental process continues to operate without the constraints of wakeful 'concentration'. From a Bergsonian perspective, despite a certain indebtedness to the past, dreaming is not simply its enslaved product, but is instead construed as one form of perception that in turn provides a particular way to condense images or to filter the image-Real that generates a subject. The very possibility of dreaming in Freud's text is instead grounded in a desire to fulfil wishes that are ultimately infantile and unconscious ones (thus the truth of the dream is ultimately to be sought in a deeply submerged or partly superseded origin). It is in this context, for Freud, that day-time psychic activity would seem to have a largely secondary significance in the formation of the dream. Indeed, he likens the remainders of conscious life, or unresolved day-time materials, to an 'entrepreneur' who unleashes the powerful 'capital' of unconscious wishes: such an 'entrepreneur' cannot 'do anything without capital; he needs a *capitalist* to take on the expenses' (p. 365). (One wonders about the seemingly unassigned role of the 'worker' in this classic scene of production, but that is perhaps by the bye here.)

The Interpretation of Dreams consequently rejects the idea that dreams are to be understood as day-facing or day-bound in the sense that they are merely a part of waking up, and that the 'time' in which they occur is exactly the same as the 'time' accompanying the process of awakening. (This idea was as popular in Freud's time as it is now.) In order to challenge this view, Freud cites those dreams in which we dream that we wake, while remaining asleep, as well as those dreams which survive or straddle brief periods of waking during the night. But in order to distinguish dreaming from waking, he is also to be found arguing that 'the first part of the dream-work is already beginning during the day' (p. 376) – that is, *before* one even sleeps, rather than simply before one wakes up. In *The Interpretation of Dreams*, then, the dream is at once 'wholly compatible with sleep' (pp. 373–4), indeed largely devoted to protecting and preserving sleep; while at the same time it is the product of long-held wishes that persist in the unconscious but which were forged during infantile waking life, and which therefore cut across day and night. ('Some experiences of my own lead me to think that the dream-work often needs more than a day and a night to deliver its results', Freud writes (p. 377).) Thus while the 'psychical system in control of the day' wishes to sleep, what happens in dreaming is merely its other side (the 'dream does continue the motivation and interests of waking life, for dream-thoughts are engaged only with what seems to be important and of great interest to us' (p. 386)). Critically, then, Freud is keen to repudiate the popular (and indeed scholarly) view that the process of dreaming is a purely 'somatic' one, caught up in forces that are simply to do with the night-time and sleep (p. 386).

In Freud's 'text' generally, therefore, the remnants of the 'day' are frequently insisted upon as of secondary importance, and they are even called 'trifling'. Indeed, their 'trifling' nature is rather important to how they function in dreaming's economy. For Freud argues that the remainders of waking life are useful and important to dreaming in the sense that they offer the unconscious 'the point of attachment it needs for transference' (p. 368). As opposed to 'the earliest and oldest of our dream-thoughts', more 'recent and trifling elements' are valuable to the dream because they 'have the least to fear from the censorship set up by resistance' (p. 367). Here, then, what is apparently 'trifling' turns out to be extremely significant and at times indispensable, precisely through its ostensible triviality. Leaving aside this important complication of the relationship between the trivial and non-trivial, however, in a still more fundamental sense the remains of the 'day' are highly non-trivial in relation to the power or activity of the unconscious to the extent that the forces which impel the dream (infantile or repressed wishes) are, as Freud insists, not purely 'somatic'. Thus he writes:

> We were able to discover in the dream-thoughts proof of highly complicated intellectual performance, operating with almost all the instrumentation of the psychic apparatus; but it still cannot be denied that these dream-thoughts originated in the day-time ... (p. 387)

The non-simple relationship of sleep and dreaming to 'day' in its double sense (i.e. both its narrow and broad sense) that we find in Freud thus sets the context for an interplay between wakefulness and slumber with which we must continue to struggle in his wake. Ultimately, for psychoanalysis, sleep is something of a double agent, since the wish to sleep on the part of the ego permits a situation whereby, during slumber itself, the capacity to hold down repressed material is reduced by a certain, inevitable relaxation of energy. While the resultant upsurge of psychic activity originating in the unconscious may not present a genuine cause for concern (the suspension of the motor function brought on by sleep renders it relatively harmless, as does a certain awareness that one is dreaming – which may result in either the continuation or termination of the dream, whichever is the more beneficial), nevertheless sleep is always, to some extent, double-facing.

Turning now to some other texts which may be located at a certain stage in Freud's career, primarily those published during the two decades after *The Interpretation of Dreams*, before *Beyond the Pleasure Principle* or *The Ego and the Id*, it is possible to trace out similar problems around the question of sleep that in fact persist in the development and refinement of his thought over the long term. Here, in particular, it is possible to see that the double-facing nature of sleep threatens to erode the power of the unconscious or at any rate the system of psychic life that is overtly proposed by psychoanalysis.

In *Jokes and their Relation to the Unconscious*,[8] from 1905, it is the dream which once more processes the day's residue of psychic activity – a 'tissue of thoughts, usually a very complicated one' – by expending its unused energy or 'interest' in a way that is 'innocuous to sleep'. This involves the construction of a wish, frequently one that is repressed in adult waking life, which may easily be fulfilled in the dream (pp. 160–1). Hence, sleep involves a double wish, as it were: first of all, the wish to sleep, which once achieved nonetheless leaves unresolved a certain 'cathexis of energy that still remains in the day's residues after it has been lowered by the state of sleep'; and, second, the fulfilment of a wish, one that often puts itself to work against the censorship imposed by waking life and which therefore arises in the context of repression (p. 165).[9] This wish-fulfilment, then, has a determining role in the formation of the dream that itself supports the wish to sleep (that is, by resisting premature awakening). One sleeps in order to occupy or attain a certain situation outside conscious life where inhibited longings can be satisfied or attemptedly resolved. But the fulfilment of such wishes serves not merely to address unconscious desires carried over from repressed waking life. It also functions to preserve the sleep that, in a particular way, consciousness wishes for – that is, by reducing or transposing the excitation that might stem from external stimuli.[10] Here then, sleep once more faces both ways. It panders to unconscious and conscious desires alike. It is difficult to know its true master, or whether indeed it has one.[11] Just a few pages further on, Freud writes that dreams 'retain their connection with the major interests of life' in that they 'occur for the sake of the one need that is active during the night – the need to sleep' (p. 179). Here, while Freud suggests that dreams serve the interests of the day as much as the appetites of the unconscious, sleep is characterized in terms of a 'need' that would seem to distinguish itself from and perhaps even transcend desire, whether conscious or unconscious. It may be that the evocation of 'need' as a term which seems to elevate itself above both conscious and unconscious wishes serves to displace the undecidable question of sleep's principal or predominating driver. In the process, however, sleep is not just reduced to a mere physiological state or condition (a 'need'), but is also paradoxically unsettled as a solid substrate or basis for the active forces at play during the formation of dreams (wish-fulfilment-repression-censorship). While it is undoubtedly by means of its function as a passive substrate that sleep is conventionally marked as purely physiological, the unresolved question of its *basis* brought on by this evocation of 'need' rather than 'desire' renders highly problematic just this attempted move or gesture towards physiological attribution that the language of 'need' would itself seem to introduce: since we cannot know its share in the *interests* underlying these different forces of the day and the night-time, or the degree to which it supports them, sleep threatens to become something as duplicitous as it is impassive. Sleep, in other words, neither simply translates the concerns of another (whether consciousness or the unconscious), nor at bottom convincingly resettles itself through recourse to the supposedly neutral concept of 'need'. And this is troubling, perhaps, for our whole attitude to sleep.

In his essay 'On Narcissism',[12] from 1914, meanwhile, Freud offers a striking analogy between illness and sleep which in fact presents the latter as less dysfunctional than one might initially expect. Here, Freud tells us that the condition of sleep 'resembles illness' to the extent that it involves a 'narcissistic withdrawal of the positions of the libido onto the subject's own self' (p. 83). Just as 'the sick man withdraws his libidinal cathexes back upon his own ego', with the result that expressions of love for another are 'suddenly replaced by complete indifference' (p. 82), so the wish to sleep entails an egoism which is unresponsive to the other, overtly at least. 'The egoism of dreams fits very well into this context', Freud remarks. (While, of course, the question of the 'other' in dreams and dreaming remains a complex issue for psychoanalysis, Freud's meaning here is perhaps better expressed in 'A Metapsychological Supplement to the Theory of Dreams',[13] from a similar period, where he writes that 'dreams are completely egoistic' in that 'the person who plays the chief part in their scenes is always to be recognized as the dreamer' (p. 223).[14])

Around this time, Freud is keen to think of sleep in terms of a certain withdrawal from the world. Thus, in 'A Metapsychological Supplement to the Theory of Dreams', he starts out by saying that, in preparation for a night's sleep, we undress our minds as much as we undress our bodies, in order to cast off all the concerns of the day. Indeed, he asserts that 'somatically, sleep is a reactivation of intra-uterine existence, fulfilling as it does the conditions of repose, warmth and exclusion of stimulus; indeed, in sleep many people assume the foetal posture'. The psychical condition of sleep is thus, we are told, characterized by a 'cessation of all interest' in the world (p. 222). By dint of this absolute retreat, sleep once more benefits not just one or other side of the 'self', but serves the ego and the libido at once. For, during night-time slumbers, a 'primitive narcissism' is offered to the ego, while the libido can hope to indulge in the 'hallucinatory satisfaction of wishes' (pp. 222–3). Indeed, Freud adds that egoism is also 'a libidinal phenomenon', and more precisely that narcissism is the name we might assign to the condition in which egoism finds itself supplemented by a 'libidinal complement' which is not merely extrinsic to it (p. 223).[15] Here, then, it is not simply a question of sleep serving two masters. Instead, sleep provides the occasion for Freud to reflect upon what seems to be a more basic narcissism in which the ego and libido coincide and are inter-implicated. This line of thinking possibly offers some resolution to the problem of sleep as both impassive and duplicitous, without-basis and complexly invested at once. Nonetheless, at the same time, Freud argues that the formation of dreams – whether in service of the ego or the libido – results not simply from a narcissistic withdrawal into 'self'. Not to be understood as merely inward-facing, dreams are also formed as a response to that which in fact *threatens* pure indulgence in this same narcissism. Such a threat comes from the residues of waking life, or a continued connection to the outside world, which dreams tackle by allying these remnants to wishes that are repressed – and which therefore may be as troubling as they are pleasurable. This assertion of dreaming as both an unrestrained flight into pure narcissism and a reaction to narcissism's limits undermines the very notion of a more basic or simple narcissism which sleep and dreaming supports, and which indeed supports dreaming and sleep. As Freud himself writes in

'A Metapsychological Supplement to the Theory of Dreams', sleep may be interrupted either by 'external stimulus' or by 'internal excitation' (p. 224): the latter, since it is both 'more obscure and more interesting' to Freud, is here given precedence. The 'internal excitation' of which Freud speaks results, once again, from the persistence of 'residues from the previous day' (these form part of the system of the preconscious), which have retained 'a certain amount of libidinal or other interest' (i.e. they somehow connect to the system of the unconscious) (p. 224).[16] As Freud had already argued in a number of previous texts, this unresolved material is precisely what prompts or activates dreaming. Thus, in 'A Metapsychological Supplement to the Theory of Dreams' dreaming is not simply a matter of indulging in the deep narcissism shared by the ego and the libido alike. It is also a matter of dealing with unreconciled psychic materials that would otherwise threaten to interrupt the narcissistic dream. Moreover, the threat to the narcissistic extravagance of dreaming which comes from the residue of the day is not simply a matter of *external* menace. Since in the case of 'internal excitation' this day-time residue acquires significance precisely to the extent that it retains a certain degree of *libidinal* interest, the dream neither stages the pure interiority of a narcissism freely at play with itself, beyond all worldly interference, nor does it serve simply to outwit dangers which remains steadfastly 'outside' narcissistic concerns. *Instead, the dream sees narcissism defending itself against its own interests.*[17] Put simply, this is what a dream is.[18]

In these terms, we might have cause to re-examine why sleep is presented as similar to illness in the psychoanalytic 'text', and yet – on the terms of the selfsame analogy by Freud – why it is also that which seeks to *defend* against sickness. Is it because narcissism is basically auto-immune that the sleep which supposedly serves and supports it is both a matter of well-being and malady, illness and health? In any event, narcissism's auto-immunity, if we may call it that, turns out to destabilize Freud's contention that sleep doesn't in fact serve two masters (and, therefore, none) by pandering to the ego and libido alike. For if the narcissism which underlies both the ego and the libido, by continually defending itself against its own interests, turns out to be a Janus-faced and indeed ultimately unmasterful master, then we return to the still-open question: on what *basis* does one sleep, and in whose *interest*? Since all physiologically oriented conceptions of sleep[19] *as well as* all theories of sleep oriented towards a subject, ego, self, consciousness, sense-perception, etc.[20] presume for this question a more or less attainable answerability (and the inter-implication of these two types of interpretation of sleep is extremely important throughout the whole philosophical discourse on this question), we might suggest once again that the reading which this Freudian 'text' provokes actually disturbs our entire outlook on sleep.

In 'A Metapsychological Supplement to the Theory of Dreams', Freud wants to describe the situation he is discussing as follows: 'the narcissism of sleep has from the outset had to admit an exception at this point, [i.e. once the problem of the day's residue is introduced – SMW] and it is here that the formation of dreams takes its start' (p. 224). Narcissism has to 'admit an exception' to itself from the 'outset'. Within a page's space, Freud is seeking 'a modification' to his 'assumption about the narcissism of sleep' on the basis that 'the theory of dream-formation ends up in a contradiction' if we assume that, during sleep, narcissism holds absolute sway. According to Freud's argument, 'the precon-scious day's residues' are 'reinforced by unconscious instinctual impulses'; but if, according to his earlier view, the latter have in fact already 'surrendered their cathexes to the ego' in the deep narcissism of sleep, then this model no longer holds up, and the process or logic whereby it happens no longer make sense (p. 225). In any event, the 'modification' Freud suggests involves questioning the idea that 'the wish to sleep that comes from the ego' is simply complied with by the unconscious (or the 'repressed portions' which inhabit its system). We are asked, now, to reject or at least challenge the idea that the ego and the forces unleashed by the unconscious take equal delight in sleep. This attempt at unravelling the knot that ties together the narcissistic ego and libido in sleep is doubtless a reaction, conscious or otherwise, to the auto-immune condition that causes Freud to admit an 'exception' to 'the narcissism of sleep' from the very 'outset'. And before long, Freud is considering not only those instances where sleep is destabilized by the strong 'instinctual cathexes' of the unconscious, but also those cases where 'the ego gives up the wish to sleep ... because of its fear of dreams' (p. 255).[21] In an extremely short space of time, then, we move from a situation in which both the ego and libido revel in slumber, to one in which Freud notes an allergic reaction to sleep which perhaps delineates the unconscious[22] as much as it threatens to haunt the ego interminably. (Before long, too, Freud is ruminating on the 'easing of communication between the *Pcs.* and the *Ucs.*' during sleep, which in fact allows a coupling together of the 'day's residues' and 'unconscious impulses' in a way that – since it amounts to a certain resistance to waking life – ends up, in fact, constituting a further 'breach in narcissism' (p. 226).) No doubt Freud's seeming volte-face concerning the relationship to narcissism of the ego/libido in sleep constitutes part of a highly unstable response to the auto-immune condition of narcissism itself; but this very same about-turn suggests that Freud's text participates in the auto-immunity with which it seeks to grapple, defending itself against itself according to the very same logic of auto-immunity that it both exposes and resists.

The future of sleep

Jacqueline Rose's essay 'On Not Being Able to Sleep: Rereading *The Interpretation of Dreams*'[23] offers an interesting commentary on the complex significance that sleep acquires within the Freudian 'text'. 'It is not easy to think about sleep. Probably because we assume that when we sleep, we relinquish our thinking selves' (p. 105), Rose begins. While *The Interpretation of Dreams* devotes itself to rescuing dreams from the easy dismissals of contemporary scientific opinion – 'to restore the dignity of the psyche to the dreamer' (p. 106), as Rose puts it – nonetheless the state or condition of sleep fosters a 'qualitatively different' form of mental life that is not easily recuperable to waking thought. If, in a footnote added more than two decades later, the dream is famously described as 'a peculiar form of thinking', still Freud's original contention is that the dream-work itself does not think – and, thus, that in both its explanation and its activity dreaming poses a fundamental challenge to thought. (It would be extremely overhasty, however, to understand Freud's two propositions as merely contradictory.) Indeed, for Rose, sleep 'breaks the line' which 'runs from the neurotic to the everyday' (p. 106), interrupting or exceeding the basic continuum that this implies by pushing the dreamer into 'hallucinatory wishful psychosis' – Freud's description of dreaming in 'A Metapsychological Supplement to the Theory of Dreams'. Here, as Rose observes, Freud implies an underlying affinity between sleep or dreaming and madness, one that spans an entire tradition of thought. As she notes, Freud himself alludes to Kant's conception of the madman as a waking dreamer. ('The lunatic is the one who dreams while awake', Freud writes in reference to Kant.) Even up to the present time, sleep scientists – frequently of the type that wish to disparage Freudian psychoanalysis altogether – still refer to dreaming as a type of psychosis. And, as we shall see, the dispute between Derrida and Foucault over the question of the 'history' of madness comes down in part to the issue of whether madness in Descartes is to be distinguished more decisively in relation to other forms of sensory error such as dreaming, as Foucault would have it, or whether, as Derrida argues, the hypothesis of dreams itself radicalizes to the most extreme point of exaggeration the hypothesis of sensory error, thus becoming, in Derrida's terms, the 'hyperbolical exasperation' of the hypothesis of madness.

Rose notes Freud's attempt, in *The Interpretation of Dreams*, to sideline the question of sleep – as distinct from that of dreaming – by labelling it merely a problem for physiology. (In the process, Freud feels justified in setting aside the entire literature on sleep – 'the only literature in the magisterial overview of the first chapter which he pays the compliment of leaving alone', as Rose wittily puts it (p. 107).) However, Rose charts the continuing presence of sleep as a problem in Freud's text. Despite Freud's own claim that he enjoys untroubled sleep, he is still to be found poring over dreams as themselves a restless reaction to the extraordinary complexity of the 'sleeping psyche'. As Rose observes: 'The psyche, one could say, never sleeps. For the interpreter of dreams, there is no sleep for sleep' (p. 107). Rose thus reads Freud's remark in *The Interpretation of Dreams* concerning the idea that one must assume 'a state of sleep for the inner life' as more of a 'plea' than a scientific proposition (p. 107). However, as soon as sleep is taken as the 'focus', writes Rose, 'fear of the dark, instead of a metaphor for the limits of knowledge, a salutary caution against psychoanalytic knowingness, turns real' (p. 109). It becomes fear itself. Indeed, it impresses itself on the mind in a way that, for Rose, resonates powerfully with one of Freud's own descriptions of dreaming. In this sense, the basic fear that psychoanalysis is forced to confront is not that of the limits to its own knowledge, but instead that of a certain regression to the night-terrors of childhood. If in *The Interpretation of Dreams*, Freud sets himself the task of building 'out into the dark', this phrase aspires to a certain sense of reassurance, combining heroic mission with technical competence (even the security of building control), only at the price of reintroducing precisely the scene of infantile dread: darkness itself. For Rose, then, psychoanalytic trepidation might not simply arise in view of its own 'crisis of knowledge' (by its very nature, such a 'crisis' invites sober, scholarly reflection, and thus calls for childhood things to be put aside). Rather, such tredipation might be little more than an expression of childhood terrors – something, indeed, which psychoanalysis may fear the most.[24] In this case, psychoanalysis would find it hard to take such fear as the simple target of its own inquiry not because of a more abstract limit set against the possibility of its own knowledge, but because the frightened child would not merely exist as the 'object' of its interest but would also constitute a projection of the very form its own experience must take. The frightened child would be both an image and expression of its fear, giving rise perhaps to merely a recurrence of that which psychoanalysis fears the most.

Rose concludes that, when thought of this way, sleep begins to look less like a 'metaphor' for some other thing, and more like a 'pathway *into*' something else (p. 110), albeit a pathway that seems relatively pathless. The task that sleep sets us, as Proust observed, is one to be accomplished with eyes closed. Rose points out that the idea of sleep as an accomplishment is at least partly misleading since, as she wants to argue, closing your eyes does not so much pave the way to sleep (as any insomniac will tell you), but instead relates properly to sleep as its 'consequence' – that is, as a symptom rather than a cause. Not everyone would agree with Rose that sleep is entirely beyond that which can be 'willed'. For there is a long tradition, from Aristotle to Nancy, that wants to associate the fall of sleep not simply with 'a loss of consciousness' but with 'the conscious plunge of consciousness into unconsciousness, which it allows to rise up in itself as it sinks down into it', as Nancy himself puts it.[25] Rose insists that sleep comes only 'inadvertently', at the point where thought strays from the idea of sleeping. This may be an extremely astute observation, though it still begs the question that it seemingly refuses to ask: namely, to what extent does 'thought' arrange for itself the conditions of its own 'fall' into sleep? Indeed, what do we mean by *thought* here? Given that for Freud the passage to dreaming leads to the onset of a 'peculiar form of thinking' that is nonetheless beyond 'thought' itself, what happens when the thought of sleep gives way – or gives itself over – to sleep 'itself'? Surely this transition is more complex than the one Rose would seem to allude to, more complex than what may be involved in the abrupt passage from insomniacal wide-awakeness to the sudden and arbitrary onslaught of sleep? By writing that 'the best way to fall asleep is to think of anything but sleep' (p. 110), Rose no doubt hints at the complexity of those relations which link 'thought' to sleep, going beyond a simple distinction between the two. (Later on in the essay, indeed, she speaks of 'the passage, the state of transition – the psychic no-man's land of waking and not waking – where Freud situates the dream' (p. 111).) Perhaps, then, the meaning of Proust's observation is deliberately ambiguous: one goes into sleep with one's eyes closed, as the accomplishment of a task to which one must remain purblind, or as the acceptance of a contract whose demands remain obscure. As Rose puts it 'we never know what will happen – or where exactly we are going – when we go to sleep' (p. 110), although doubtless we still go into this situation with our eyes (partly) open. Unlike the one who swoons or is involuntarily asphyxiated, we wish for sleep, we consciously pursue unconsciousness, we build into the unknown. In a seeming contradiction of interests, we want as much as we fear the dark. (This 'want' is perhaps what gives the dark its very edge.)

As Rose notes, perhaps Freud sought to relinquish psychoanalysis's 'want' and 'fear' of sleep at the point hypnosis was abandoned as an analytic technique. If hypnosis aims to 'suspend the patient ... at sleep's threshold' (just the point of complexity at which mental life remains irreducible either to unflinching wide-awakeness or to the onslaught of an absolutely unknowable repose – a complexity, indeed, which may perhaps pertain *whenever* one is asleep or awake), then the discontinuation of hypnosis suggests the attempt to 'let go' of sleep, as Rose puts it (p. 111). To let it 'go' as a psychoanalytic concern in its own right, or in other words to divorce the problems confronted by the analysand and analyst alike from the experience or condition of sleep per se. Of course, the very combination of 'fear' and 'want' involved in psycho-analysis's relationship to the 'dark' means that such an abandonment is, more generally, impossibly fated. Once again, the whole episode looks like another case of psychoanalysis seeking to defend against its own interests.

In this context, it is apt that Rose mentions Freud's recounting of a dream, the night after attending a funeral, where he encounters an enigmatic sign: 'You are requested to close the eyes' (cited in Rose, p. 111). As Freud himself observes, the legend conveys a double and deeply ambiguous meaning: one should remain vigilant concerning one's duty to the dead, one should be alive and awake to such a duty; but also, one should perform this duty oneself, close one's own eyes as if one were dead. Such a double meaning expresses nothing less, perhaps, than the curious and complex condition of mental life while asleep. (One should remain observant of, and alive to, the spectre of death that continually haunts the dreamer; indeed, one *must* do as much, since dreams mark nothing less than death's limit, resisting as they do the passage to total sleep and thus death itself. And yet, as Proust remarks, if sleep is a task, it is one we accomplish with our eyes closed.) But this double meaning applies also to psychoanalysis itself, which builds out to the dark with a trepidation and longing born of 'fear' and 'want', recalling and replaying childhood terrors which involve revulsion and recoil at the thought (or the fantasy) of closing the eyes of the dead, as much as consternation and curiosity at the thought of one's own drooping lids. Indeed, as Rose suggests, the legend divides psychoanalysis in its very history, split uneasily as it is between 'a psychoanalysis which sees its task as waking the soul into reason' – thus, perhaps, closing the eyes of the dead – 'and a psychoanalysis which does not know, cannot be sure, whether it is itself awake' (p. 112). Divides the psychoanalytic ego,[26] that is to say, as perhaps just another divided 'ego' among others.

The vexed relation of the problem of sleep to that of the recursive image – and experience – of childhood is, as may now be obvious, central to Rose's essay. For her, a key question for Freud – the father of six whose own child refused to be bed-ridden even by the most troubling fever – is whether the child sleeps. Or whether, in fact, the passage to sleep and dreams only reawakens the child, bringing it (back) to life – as in the famous dream of the burning child that continues to haunt readers of *The Interpretation of Dreams*. Every dream, suggests Freud, gives expression to infantile wishes; or, to put it as Rose does, every dream includes, for psychoanalysis, 'the wish *for* infancy' (p. 115) (which may remain, nonetheless, an *adult* wish).

But how far does this wish go? In *The Interpretation of Dreams*, Freud notes that sometimes his patients parody him by going in search of memories studded with interest or importance – memories, however, characterized foremost by their seeming absurdity – by looking back beyond their very earliest years to, as Freud puts it, a 'time when they were *not yet in the land of the living*' (cited in Rose, p. 118). As Rose notes, this apparent send-up may not be so crazy. 'For if the part of the mind which travels back ... is unconscious to us', she writes, 'how can we possibly be sure, when we sleep, where it might take us, just how far back in fact we go?' (p. 118). Rose cites Proust's idea that each of us is possessed of, and is in fact constituted by, memories we cannot recall, memories which may therefore be said to extend beyond the reach of the life presently lived. Thus, for Proust, the unrecalled time before birth is to the living man what his own life may become for whatever he is destined to be after death. Such time is bound to be unremembered, but for all that the question of its significance cannot be too hastily dismissed. Such thinking extends psychoanalysis somewhat beyond itself, argues Rose, pointing to moments in the Freudian 'text' where this begins to happen. Psychic reality, as Freud himself once noted, may not be limited to one form of existence, and in its strange particularity, its plasticity, its complex determinacy, should not be confused with a simple idea of '*material* reality'. Dreams as the repositories of an unrecollected body of memories may therefore point backward to a radical infancy, one that even goes before or beyond infancy itself. Yet Rose wants to insist that they are also 'generative, forward-looking, not in the predictable but unpredictable sense':

> Precisely because they lead us back into the deepest recesses of the psyche – to the point where for Proust the psyche goes beyond the psyche – they lead forward into something else. (p. 121)

Here, dreams not only complicate – and perhaps unravel – the narcissistic 'self', but also stretch far beyond the dispositions of an 'ego' or subject, constitutively supplementing our present life and, for that matter, any conception of 'life' construed in terms of a metaphysics of presence. And, through her rereading of *The Interpretation of Dreams*, this conception of dreaming on Rose's part – rather than simply reasserting an unknowable past which defines us all – devotes itself to the prospect of a future which cannot be prophesied. A future without easy reassurances to dream of in the dark. Here, unmasterable sleep, facing in more than one direction (or, rather, more and less than one), leads us out to who knows where. Undecidably split between sickness and well-being, security and risk, wakefulness and the dark, sleep takes us to that threshold where – however impossibly – we defend against our own interests, and seek to overcome them. Such a threshold is at once a site of potential disintegration; but it is also, as Rose points out, one of transformation, right from the beginning, perhaps before any 'beginning', at any rate always beginning again, always still to come.

Phenomenology of Sleep

Husserl: Being asleep, falling asleep

Can phenomenology have anything to say about sleep? In a recent essay, Nicolas de Warren has tried to suggest ways in which Jean-Luc Nancy's insistence that there is no phenomenology of sleep may lack nuance in relation to Husserlian thought.[1] As his argument unfolds, Warren points out: 'Husserl's analysis of time-consciousness is centered on the exemplary phenomenon of the perceptual apprehension of the time-object' (p. 276). An obvious example here is that of melody, which is composed of a succession of individual notes – each of their own time-duration – that follow or precede one another within a sequence that allows for the appreciation of unified, melodic form only on the basis of retention (retaining what has gone before as a condition of one's experience of the present) and protention (a projection or expectation of what is to come that remains essential to how the 'now' is to be understood). In the appreciation of melody, we pass over from now to now, as Husserl puts it, although in a to-and-fro movement which includes the future as much as the past (what is still to come as much as what has gone before) that remains intrinsic to the experience of melody as it impresses itself upon us 'now', in each fleeting instant. As de Warren puts it, 'every original presentation ... becomes necessarily modified in a retentional consciousness' of what has passed but still remains essential in its sequencing with the present; while, at the same time, 'every retentional modification of an original presentation motivates a protentional consciousness that ... anticipates a now-phase yet to come' (p. 277). Thus, argues de Warren, the 'living presence' of the present – the 'now' in its immediacy – depends on a profound 'de-presen-tification', to use Husserl's term, through which a constitutive absence (though not simply an absence *as such*) defines the very possibility of the experience of presence. Hence, the past – as a 'just-past' – deeply informs our consciousness of the 'now', and yet what has gone before is also bound to sink away somewhat (as increasingly a 'far' rather than 'near retention') as the present continues to reconstitute itself going forward. Crucially, as de Warren observes, 'Husserl metaphorically characterizes this transformation of retention' from near to far 'as a shift from *falling asleep* to *being asleep*' (pp. 280–1). While 'far' retentions are akin to the past's gradual immersion in a deeper sleep, near retention looks much more like a finely balanced 'falling asleep', construed as a profound movement of unconsciousness within consciousness, one which conveys the constitutive impact upon consciousness itself of that which is not immediately present to consciousness. Since this 'self-forgetting, or *falling asleep*, of consciousness is original to the self-constitution of time-consciousness' (pp. 281–2), the living present is just a feature of the basic time-consciousness that is itself constituted by an originary difference between a certain wakefulness and a certain falling asleep. However, the latter – falling asleep – does not impose itself in extrinsic fashion, it does not intrude from the outside; rather, it is intrinsic to the very possibility of wakefulness itself. As de Warren puts it, constituted 'in its metaphorical meaning as "falling asleep," the retentional modification of consciousness fixes the sense in which consciousness still has itself – retains itself – without being conscious or awake to itself', i.e. without having access in an immediate present to that which would appear to constitute its immediate present (pp. 282–3). Indeed, this disposition of consciousness in terms of time-consciousness implies that wakefulness should be construed in terms of a wide openness to experience, by means of which attentiveness to a particular object is just a delimited manifestation (in fact the former could never be reduced to the latter). Perhaps most strikingly, however, de Warren's reading of Husserl suggests interesting ways to think the idea that one is never entirely awake, that a certain sleep in fact makes possible wakefulness itself.

Merleau-Ponty: 'There is a moment when sleep "comes" … and I succeed in becoming what I was trying to be'

In part one of *Phenomenology of Perception*, in a section entitled 'The Body in its Sexual Being', Merleau-Ponty writes:

For the dreamer, indeed, who is far removed from the language of the waking state, this or that genital excitation or sexual drive *is* without more ado this image of a wall being climbed or cliff-face being scaled ... The dreamer's penis *becomes* the serpent which appears in the obvious content. What we have just said about the dreamer applies equally to that ever slumbering part of ourselves which we feel to be anterior to our representations, to that individual haze through which we perceive the world. There are here blurred outlines, distinctive relationships which are in no way 'unconscious' ...[2]

The principal aim of this part of the book is to inquire how 'we bring into existence, for ourselves' a world – more specifically, space, the body, the object, the instrument. Wanting to 'bring to light the birth of being for us' beyond our relationship to the natural world – which presents itself as existing 'over and above its existence for me' – Merleau-Ponty turns to the 'affective life'. An investigation of how 'significance and reality' is produced for us, by us, may, he argues, assist our understanding of 'how things and beings can exist in general' (pp. 154–5). In particular, it is the study of sexual life that gives direction to Merleau-Ponty's concerns in this chapter.

Concentrating on the case study of a man who, after suffering 'a wound of limited extent in the occipital region', seems to lose all interest in sexual activity, Merleau-Ponty suggests that the physical injury itself is not enough to explain this loss of desire; rather, it is 'the very structure of perception or erotic experience which has undergone change' in him (p. 156). What has been lost, or rather what has changed, is the once-desirous perception of another's body, 'subtended' as it was by an always individualized 'sexual schema', one which included the very 'gestures' of the desiring body itself. For Merleau-Ponty, then, the 'subject' as much as the 'object' becomes 'integrated' into what he calls the 'emotional totality' of this structure of perception. In the case of the man in question, however, perception has 'lost its erotic structure', both in spatial and temporal terms. Or, as Merleau-Ponty puts it: 'What has disappeared from the patient is his power of projecting before himself a sexual world, of putting himself in an erotic situation', or of maintaining such a situation for himself (p. 156).

From this, Merleau-Ponty suggests that erotic or sexual life is maintained according to a structure of perception which is not based purely in 'consciousness' (construed in terms of a disembodied 'mind'), but rather one which depends on an embodied integration in the scene of desire. The sexual life, in other words, relies on an ability to, as it were, 'throw' oneself bodily into the complex schemas connected to eroticized 'perception'. Thus, he writes:

> A sight has a sexual significance for me, not when I consider, even confusedly, its possible relationship to the sexual organs or to pleasurable states, but when it exists for my body … (p. 157)

One does not, therefore, realize or experience one's desire principally in terms of its 'mental' understanding (and one can no more comprehend it by way of abstract thought or intellection). Whereas the very process of 'mental' comprehension would tend to subsume the experience under an 'idea' with which it could never be fully integrated, desire maintains itself through a 'body to body' connection which is itself integral to the structure of perception through which the sexual life arises. Far from reducing sexuality to a bodily function, this conception of affectivity reconnects 'body' and 'mind' without seeking to establish an order of priority, and by resisting falling back into the entire ensemble of dualisms which help to construct their supposed difference.

Thus, Merleau-Ponty observes that the man of the case study in question is characterized not simply by a loss of sexual interest, but by an emotional neutrality more generally, a detached and abstract relationship to the world, a mechanical and decisionistic rather than intuitive engagement with all that surrounds him. These personal characteristics are not, however, just the products of a certain attitude of mind; instead, they reflect a particular disposition of the body – or rather a certain failing of embodiment – in the world. From this, Merleau-Ponty writes:

> We discover both that sexual life is one more form of original intentionality, and also bring to view the vital origins of perception, motility and representation by basing all these 'processes' on an 'intentional arc' which gives way in the patient, and which, in the normal subject, endows experience with its degree of vitality and fruitfulness. (p. 157)

Hence, sexuality is neither a special case, nor the original example or template, of what characterizes human existence. Rather, it opens onto the entirety of the active, cognitive being. While such an argument would seem to suggest possible disagreements with the psychoanalytic understanding of sexuality (i.e. its determining originality for Freud), Merleau-Ponty is nevertheless quick to herald psychoanalysis's achievements in reintegrating sexuality into the human being without locating sexual attitudes, preferences or desires simply in 'consciousness' and, equally, without reducing psychology to biology, anatomy or physiognomy. In other words, he celebrates what he terms a psychoanalytic 'dialectic' that relates body and mind in more complex ways, and thereby suggests that even Freudian psychoanalysis may not be entirely opposed to 'the phenomenological method' (p. 158), instead giving it another opportunity for development (as is the case here).

Merleau-Ponty thus describes Freud's understanding of the 'sexual' as not limited to reproductive, instinctual or genital 'ends' (nor, for Merleau-Ponty, would the 'sexual' be the product of the unconscious as distinct from the generality of one's – embodied – phenomenal being). Rather, for Merleau-Ponty, Freudian 'sexuality' is but an expression of 'the general power' of the 'psychosomatic subject': namely, that of 'taking root in different settings, of establishing himself through different experiences'. Sexuality, in other words, is simply a way or means of projecting one's 'manner of being towards the world' or, indeed, *in* the world (p. 158). Accordingly, when properly understood, the 'sexual symptoms at the root of all neuroses' only 'symbolize a whole attitude'. To recast the psychoanalytic interpretation of sexuality, then, human life may only 'rest on' sexuality, as Merleau-Ponty puts it, to the extent that sexuality must itself be understood in terms of 'the elaboration of a general form of life' (p. 158). Again, psychoanalysis's achievement in generalizing 'sexuality' is foregrounded here, and its notion of an entire 'sexual substructure of life' is reinterpreted in these terms.

Merleau-Ponty continues to develop this engagement with psychoanalytic thought. On the basis of the argument that he wants to elaborate, it therefore becomes misleading to proclaim that all facets of life have a decidedly 'sexual' significance, for this would be to determine the 'sexual' according to a restricted sense or meaning that his own approach refuses to recognize. Equally, it might be just as misleading to interpret every 'sexual phenomenon' in terms of some larger 'existential significance', if existence is thereby construed as a somehow grander condition onto which sexuality merely opens a small window, or towards which it clears a narrow pathway. Sexuality is not merely a particular 'expression' of being, an 'epiphenomenon', or a simple 'reflection' of a certain disposition of existence. Rather, it is a *manner* of being, the manner which being has (regardless of whether one is sexually active or competent, or not – as this text proceeds, Merleau-Ponty is anxious to disentangle the precise character of one's sexual performances more overtly from the question of one's manner of being in the world).

Existence is thus always embodied, and sexuality constitutes itself neither as the closely defined origin of all embodied experience, nor however as a mere subset of the generality of lived bodily life to which it gives expression. Instead, the entirety of embodied life, which sexuality pervades in one way or another without necessarily dominating as such, provides the context for understanding the complex reciprocity of the 'psyche' and the 'flesh' outside of established orders of priority (such as those which elevate 'spirit' over 'matter' or perhaps contrariwise the 'real' over the 'imitation' or representation – although of course what relates these two dualisms is never just a matter of reversal).

At this point in the discussion, as if to clarify further his arguments by dint of a specific illustration, Merleau-Ponty turns to another case study, that of a young girl whose mother has forbidden her contact with her lover. As a consequence, the girl loses the ability to sleep, to eat, and, ultimately, to speak. As it turns out, she had in fact lost the power of speech on more than one occasion in the past, due to the trauma of an earthquake and subsequently because of a 'severe fright'. Merleau-Ponty observes that a more 'strictly Freudian interpretation' of the story would draw attention to 'the oral phase of sexual development' that would once more seem to be in question here. However, he argues that what gets 'fixated' on the mouth is not just 'sexual' in character, but has to do more generally with a refusal to communicate, to correspond or co-exist with others. In fact, the girl's symptoms suggest a 'break with life itself'. She will no more ingest and process the events and circumstances of her life, than the food she would normally eat. Her aphonia replays the traumatic reaction to perceived threats of death during childhood, aggressively phasing out all others in order that she might devote herself solely to 'her own personal fate' (p. 161). Loss of speech throws her back upon the past, allowing her to deal with – or, rather, avoid – the present crisis by reverting solipsistically to 'her favourite forms of behaviour', rather than confronting the future to which her mother has condemned her. Indeed, her loss of speech represents a rejection of human society that is all the more profound, since to all appearances it is 'involuntary' rather than the result of a planned refusal to form words or use language, which would still of course deliberately convey a 'message' to the world. (Interestingly, Merleau-Ponty does not offer an explicit interpretation of the meaning of the girl's insomnia, although presumably this could be put down to a refusal to refresh herself in preparation for the coming days – a reaction just as world-averse as that of the catatonic.)

While Merleau-Ponty broadens the interpretation of this case study beyond its narrowly sexual meanings, nevertheless he is quick to add that the girl's physical symptoms do not convey some 'existential' or 'mental' crisis in the way that 'stripes indicate rank, or a house-number a house'. 'The sick girl', he writes, 'does not mime with her body a drama played out "in her consciousness". By losing her voice she does not present a public version of an "inner state"' (p. 161). Her aphonia is not 'a deliberate or voluntary silence' (if it were, its meaning would be altogether different, though perhaps no less the sign of ailment), but is instead a product of the embodied life's manner of being in the world, this time in the context of what is too narrowly understood as 'psychic' disorder (which nevertheless connects to her life more generally). Moreover, notwithstanding the psychoanalytic elements of Merleau-Ponty's interpretation, the girl's loss of speech is not simply evidence of the forces of the *unconscious* unleashed afresh by the present crisis. Rather, her reaction represents a certain reversion to a manner of being in the world learnt or developed in childhood on just the basis Merleau-Ponty has been describing. As such, the loss of memory, say, is no more simply an effect of the unconscious than it is a conscious decision:

> Thus, in hysteria and repression, we may well overlook something although we know of it, because our memories and our body, instead of presenting themselves to us in singular and determinate conscious acts, are enveloped in generality. Through this generality we still have them, but just enough to hold them at a distance from us. (p. 162)

The ambivalent relation of 'having' and 'not having' our memories is not, then, the product of some interminable struggle between the unconscious and the conscious mind, but is instead a sort of compromise fashioned from the disparate resources stretched out across the 'generality' of embodied life. The chances of remembering and, indeed, of forgetting are forged in just this embodied 'generality', and nowhere else. In fact, the deeply questionable possibility of ever switching off or stepping outside this 'generality' may be imagined only through its resurgence in another form: 'a night's sleep', says Merleau-Ponty, is an 'anonymous' or anonymizing force only to the extent that it may surmount that which is 'of the same nature as it' (p. 163). Sleep, then, which had received no specific interpretation in terms of the case of the love-struck girl, now returns in the very image of 'the general form of life' that determines being's embodiment in the world. Neither driven nor dominated by consciousness, nor confined to merely physical causes or bodily functions, this 'general form of life' is no more the product or expression of a 'waking mind' than it is the upshot of insensible material forces. Instead, it plays on the cusp of the two, reconstituting each according to a certain 'dialectic' under way, the logic of which – while it would seem to be synthetic – nonetheless results in a series of examples which dwell on what is anomalous and dysfunctional, on what continually misfires in an unstintingly embodied psychodynamics. Be that as it may, the fact that just such a 'general form of life' might possibly be 'surmounted' only by the equivalent 'power' of sleep – which therefore serves as something of its mirror-image – suggests that Merleau-Ponty considers sleep to be the closest thing you can get to ... well, life itself. Or, that it provides as good a name as any for the strange and complex way in which we are immersed in life 'itself'.

Returning to the case of a 'lost' voice (as illustrative of what occurs in a number of other maladies), Merleau-Ponty returns to the theme that such a loss must happen below the level of the 'will'. Consequently, effective treatment of the condition may not depend upon making the patient 'aware of the origin of his illness' (another departure from psychoanalysis, perhaps), but may in fact rely on some input that occurs below the level of consciousness:

> ... sometimes the touch of a hand puts a stop to the spasms and restores the patient to his speech and the same procedure, having acquired a ritual signifi-cance, will subsequently be enough to deal with fresh attacks. In any case, in psychological treatment of any kind, the coming to awareness would remain purely cognitive, the patient would not accept the meaning of his disturbances as revealed to him without the personal relationship to the doctor, or without the confidence and friendship felt towards him, and the change of existence resulting from this friendship. (p. 163)

Once more, one's psychic condition is not just dependent on the strength of the conscious mind (or the success one has had in tackling the unconscious), but comes down to the specifics of embodied being in the world. The cure, like the symptom, may therefore be sought below the level of consciousness (which is nevertheless not that of the 'unconscious' in the sense conventionally attributed to psychoanalysis). This is perhaps the more immediate meaning, or at any rate the context for the meaning, of Merleau-Ponty's earlier, rather enigmatic evocation of sleep: a symptom may be eased by a treatment which is not itself an expression of reason's triumph, in just the same way that a night's sleep has the power to overcome or improve 'involuntary' disorders, though it itself is a somewhat involuntary activity occurring – like the ailment it alleviates – below the level of the 'will'.

Then, at last, Merleau-Ponty comes back to sleep in a more explicit, or perhaps less enigmatic, way. He compares the loss of voice which has so fascinated him to sleep itself (permit me to quote at length):

> I lie down in bed ... with my knees drawn up; I close my eyes and breathe slowly, putting my plans out of my mind. But the power of my will or consciousness stops there. As the faithful, in the Dionysian mysteries, invoke the god by miming scenes from his life, I call up the visitation of sleep by imitating the breathing and posture of the sleeper. The god is actually there when the faithful can no longer distinguish themselves from the part they are playing, when their body and their consciousness cease to bring in, as an obstacle, their particular opacity, and when they are totally fused in the myth ... sleep 'comes', settling on this imitation of itself which I have been offering to it, and I succeed in becoming what I was trying to be: an unseeing and almost unthinking mass, riveted to a point in space and in the world henceforth only through the anonymous alertness of the senses. It is true that this last link makes waking up a possibility: through these half-open doors things will return or the sleeper will come back into the world ... In this sense the sleeper is never completely isolated within himself, never totally a sleeper, and the patient is never totally cut off from the intersubjective world, never totally ill. But what, in the sleeper and the patient, makes possible a return to the real world, are still only impersonal functions, sense organs and language. We remain free in relation to sleep and sickness to the exact extent to which we remain always involved in the waking and healthy state, our freedom rests on being in a situation, and is itself a situation. Sleep and waking, illness and health are not modalities of consciousness or will, but presuppose an 'existential step'. (p. 164)

Once more, doesn't sleep look uncannily like, or rather open uncannily onto, the 'general form of life' that Merleau-Ponty is at such pains to describe? Doesn't sleep emerge, here, as the strange double of being's embodiment in the world, the mirror-image of life 'itself'? The idea of a body 'riveted to a point in space and in the world henceforth only through the anonymous alertness of the senses' comes close enough to a description of the conditions of embodied perception (i.e. perception not governed in the last instance by a detached or transcendent consciousness) that it makes waking up – wakefulness itself – a 'possibility'. Consciousness, indeed, only imitates being, miming the 'posture' or embodied situation of the sleeper by an act of will that is destined to come up short.[3] The moment when sleep 'comes', 'settling on this imitation of itself which I have been offering to it, and I succeed in becoming what I was trying to be' thus marks the limit of consciousness, at the very same time that it opens onto a more fundamental 'situation' of life. (One only truly invokes the god at the point where the faithful 'no longer distinguish themselves from the part they are playing', where the distinction between the imitation and its more original or authentic origin is lost.) It is as if, in order to reconstitute an 'intersubjective' connection to the 'real world' – a connection that is no more fully mastered by consciousness in waking life than it is wholly abandoned during sleep, since even sleep puts us into an embodied 'situation' in the world – being relies on 'impersonal functions' ('sense organs and language') which are themselves possible only on condition of a 'situation' of which consciousness is more the effect than the cause. Whether asleep or awake, our state or condition depends upon this 'situation' first and foremost. As such, wakefulness and slumber are not 'modalities of consciousness', says Merleau-Ponty. Instead, consciousness and sleep alike are expressions of a more fundamental 'situation' of existence – to which, however, one would seem to draw closer in the passage from wakefulness to sleep. Indeed, within the space of just a few lines, Merleau-Ponty is to be found suggesting that the withdrawal from everyday life is not merely an expression of existential disorder (aphonia) or a certain privation of consciousness (sleep), but that it also represents the deeper desire to 'shut myself up in this anonymous life which subtends my personal one'. This would seem to look something like a necessarily partial and temporary self-enclosure, although it in fact dissolves towards a more radical anonymity at the root of being. That said, enclosing oneself in this 'anonymous life' simultaneously reinvigorates the possibility of carrying on, in that it also 'opens me out upon the world and places me in a situation there'. But, by and large, such reinvigoration happens not because of 'an intellectual effort or by an abstract decree of the will', but through a 'concentrated effort' or 'genuine gesture' of the body, through which, Merleau-Ponty adds, it 'acquires significance beyond itself' (pp. 164–5).

Returning to the question of aphonia as a key illustration of his thinking, then, Merleau-Ponty argues that it is not a refusal of life which occurs with the loss of one's voice, since this is but a specific reaction that takes shape within embodied life in its 'generality'. It is not life, therefore, but only 'others', or a future beyond our control or experience, that are rejected in these circumstances (this rejection is, for the most part, necessarily partial and therefore frequently temporary, he suggests). Thus, through aphonia the body 'transforms ideas into things', just as the body does in the situation of sleep, turning 'mimicry of sleep' into 'real sleep', therefore actualizing existence in a certain way. Merleau-Ponty writes: 'The body can symbolize existence because it brings it into being and actualizes it' (p. 164) – although the use of the word 'symbolize' here obviously complicates matters, at the very least suggesting once more that Merleau-Ponty wants to avoid the impression of reducing existence to merely bodily functions. 'In so far as it carries within it "sense organs", bodily existence is never self-sufficient ... it continually sets the prospect of living before me', he says; 'I never quite become a thing in the world' (p. 165). Or, again: 'The body expresses total existence, not because it is an external accompaniment to that existence, but because existence comes into its own in the body' (p. 166). To this extent, our dualistic conception of 'body' and 'mind' amounts to an artificial anatomy which misses the true nature of being in the world.

Through its focus on the sexual being of the body (which indeed goes far beyond the question of sexuality itself), Merleau-Ponty's phenomenology of perception makes of sleep as much a feature of our being in the world as wakefulness itself. Indeed, since it is the 'situation' of sleep, perhaps more than anything else, that would seem to allow for 'the elaboration of a general form of life', sleep for Merleau-Ponty looks less like the last stop before death, and more like the very passage opening onto existence,[4] understood as the anonymous ground of our personal lives.

The Dream about the Dream

Some basic elements, to begin with: Celan's 'Edgar Jené and The Dream About The Dream',[1] from the late 1940s, concerning Jené, surrealist painter. First of all, there is the one who says: 'I am supposed to tell you some of the words I heard deep down in the sea' as 'I followed Edgar Jené beneath his paintings' (p. 3); second, perhaps, a mouth that speaks, as it had done during sleep, moving ahead; also, in the midst of this, an exchange over Kleist's *Marionette Theatre*. Three (doubtless more than three, more or less than three) parts, components, elements in play.

The mouth shifts, it becomes dislocated, though emboldened for 'having often spoken in my sleep' (p. 4). It is transplanted, 'placed higher than my eyes' (p. 3). It moves up and onward, goes ahead of itself, speaks ahead of itself, laughing in the face that once was its own, speaking against, *right up against* this other one it will have been, perhaps: '"Well, old identity-monger, what did you see and recognize, you brave doctor of tautology?"' (p. 4). In the tragicomedy of naming, the tautological circle repeats and opens itself, namelessly. As the mouth speaks above and ahead of itself.

So close to the beginning, so near the shoreline, the 'sea's mirror surface' (p. 3) at last bursts open, granting unguided passage across a path-ridden, hence pathless, universe. Footfalls fall in ungrounded flight, someone makes way. It is 'strenuous' (p. 3). What encourages the 'absolute *naïveté*' which dreams of turning 'simple words' into pure names (p. 4)? It is a dream. Ornately constructed. It dreams of shaking the foundations of a world already left behind, a world of 'evil and injustice': namely, a world of 'lies' (p. 4). Lies exposed and exorcised, so that they may be left behind. As the emboldened mouth, lost in dreams perhaps (perhaps heading a different way), once more breaks apart, opening around and against itself again.

Who dreams this? Who pursues this dream? Who treads the lip of a surface that folds and breaks against itself, the deep interiority that is dreamt of beneath, still pressing against the shimmering edge of this outside which crashes down, time and again? Who wishes to 'follow Edgar Jené beneath his paintings' (p. 3)?

Is it the one still above the surface, the one found at the text's shore? The inaugural or inaugurating one, who – before the membrane is even torn – wearily declares: 'I am supposed to tell you some of the words I heard deep down in the sea where there is so much silence and so much happens'? (p. 3). (As if the exertion to come had already taken its toll? As if the dream's journey had already been left behind? As if the end and the beginning might at last coalesce only as the expression of a certain exhaustion?) Or is it, instead, the mouth – this other one, 'placed higher than the eyes', going ahead of itself, speaking above itself, against itself, but still going onwards, over itself, down beneath?

Whether this mouth or the other one, a conversation with a friend is remembered, one having once spoken to the other, it seems. Concerning Kleist's *Marionette Theatre*, where the puppet – *so it is said* – acquires a grace denied to human beings. Consciousness, self-consciousness, breaks nature apart. Reflection divides the world. Man is left on the shores of an ocean that dazzles and blinds, an ocean scorched by bright sunlight which redoubles as if in a vast looking glass. The eye that catches and casts light is itself caught in the reflective glare. It closes and opens. Thought and feeling separate, combine, differ. Kleist's *Marionette Theatre* speaks, though, of an original simplicity before or beyond this impasse, of the chance of a crossing to the other side, or back again to the origin, borne perhaps by an 'absolute *naïveté* ... purified of the slag of centuries of hoary lies about the world' (p. 4), as Celan's text puts it. Or, rather, one voice speaks of this, another not. (Reflecting, perhaps, the conversation that was supposedly once had, between the 'friend' and the other, concerning the *Marionette Theatre* itself.) The uncompromised grace of the inhuman creature is bandied in a puppet show. But still, only art can stage the dream, the vision of the journey, the possibility of a crossing or a return. As such, the artificiality of its reflective contours is marked with overwhelming irony. Infinity caught in a hall of mirrors, identity with the absolute broken off by the expression of its possibility. The shimmering edge of the surface not just shattered but newly reflected in the depths of our dreams.

'How could one regain that original grace?' asks Celan's text (p. 4). The reply is staged, in the mouth of the 'friend', as follows: 'It was, my friend held, by letting reason purify our unconscious inner life that we could recapture the immediacy of the beginning – which would in the end give meaning to our life and make it worth living' (p. 4). The possibility of a ring-shaped world, a returning coalescence of beginning and end which, already, has come to look exhausted. Double irony – that of the ironic repetition (or return) of an already worn-out possibility, and that of the obvious puppetry of the friend's inserted interjection.

Celan's text would therefore seem to ridicule without remorse the 'absolute *naïveté*' of which it had spoken, by putting words into another's mouth – neither the mouth of the one 'who is supposed to tell you some of the words I heard deep down in the sea', nor the mouth 'placed higher than my eyes'. But this third 'mouth' – the mouth of the 'friend' whose discourse is devoted to such lofty concerns – speaks nonetheless in a puppet theatre, which, if it does not merely revolve around the other two, undoubtedly orchestrates itself so as to stage (and indeed to suspend or 'string up') the relations of these two, including the possible relationship between their linguistic performances. By so doing, the text thus keeps radically open the question: 'Who speaks?' The third voice, that of the 'friend', does not speak in its own right; instead, it is inserted somewhat ventriloquistically into the text. And the concerns of the 'friend' form part of the concerns that are already 'on-stage', precisely. The contrivance of the friend's identification with the 'idealist' interlocutor in Kleist's text only replays the concerns which Celan's writing performs in 'Edgar Jené and The Dream About The Dream'. By voicing the dream without which the text could not open itself *even as an ironic performance of such a dream*, the friend is not merely an outsider with whom the entire scenography of the text might dispense. In other words, the friend's dream of immediacy, eternity, purity and renewal cannot be set aside without compunction, since it constitutes part of the ironic performance that gives to the other(s) an inaugurating possibility.

The friend's naïvely 'Kleistian' dream, in which 'true (primitive) meaning' (p. 5) is given back to words as the privileged expression of a return to the constancy of a ring-shaped world, nevertheless draws a 'first objection', an objection from the first:

> It was simply this: I knew that anything that happened was more than an addition to the given, more than an attribute more or less difficult to remove from the essence, that it changed the essence in its very being and thus cleared the way for ceaseless transformation. (p. 5)

The project of purifying 'the slag of centuries of hoary lies about the world', of overcoming the world's division by restoring the primordiality of a pure language, is thus undone by the fact that the possibility of an (altering) repetition is already inscribed at the origin, as a condition of inauguration. This cannot be overcome, simply or otherwise. From the beginning, *anything that may happen* enters into the very possibility of the 'essence' or the 'given', changing it, transforming it, right from the outset. The uniqueness of an original world or word, its irreplaceable event, remains a singular occurrence to the extent that it makes its incision, inscribes itself, manifests itself, *on condition of* an always possible re-marking. Even that which is most 'original' is not, therefore, simply a pure, ring-shaped form, self-containing, self-sufficient; it is always already repeatable, or, better still, iterable, since every repetition (*iter* – 'again') inevitably alters (*itara* – 'other'), an irreducible heteronomy that goes all the way down to the bottom. Unfathomable. The very signature of a constant world, even in its most singular untranslatability, would remark itself, validate itself, establish its trait, on condition of its possible inscription at another time or in another place – an 'other' which could not simply restitute itself to some prior 'essence' or 'origin' since it would instead provide the very conditions of possibility for what is originally 'given'. From the first word, this possibility inhabits the ring-shaped world of 'simple words', takes possession of it, makes it go ahead of itself, speak above itself and against itself, *right against itself*. And each word, all language, every text commemorates itself in just this way. Each anniversary comes to pass, not simply by way of the annular motif, the figure of the ring ('so that tomorrow could again be yesterday', as the friend would have it). Each anniversary also opens onto an unknowable future, an uncontainable repetition still to come. (Whether or not the latter might have foreseen it, Derrida will come to speak of Celan's writings in just these terms.[2])

'"Well, old identity-monger, what did you see and recognize, you brave doctor of tautology?"': the mouth shifts, it becomes dislocated, though emboldened for 'having often spoken in my sleep'. Transplanted, 'placed higher than my eyes', it goes ahead of itself, speaks above itself, against itself, still going onwards, over itself, down beneath, following Edgar Jené beneath his paintings, in the midst of the dream about the dream, which transforms as it repeats, the irony of return.

Against the 'sea's mirrored surface' which beguiles or bedazzles the 'I' that inaugurates the text, the 'friend' invokes instead a shining 'sun of justice' (p. 5). This, in order to reproach his interlocutor, and to stick stubbornly to his 'Kleistian' dream. Unlike those sun-rays that redouble in the vast looking glass of the sea's surface, the 'sun of justice' permits the ocean's depth and darkness to be fathomed – and thus, to be raised up – by 'reason' alone (in fact, in the discourse of the 'friend', the sea's 'dark springs' are transformed into a 'well' or veritable wellspring of reason (p. 5)). Celan – if it is indeed he – responds to this rebuke in the following way: 'I saw that this reproach was aimed at my professing that, since we know the world and its institutions are a prison for man and his spirit, we must do all we can to tear down its walls' (p. 5). Here, the text draws on another 'Kleist' of the *Marionette Theatre*: since it is inevitably a vision or dream, the ring-shaped world which would seem to make possible a return to the original order of things risks re-setting the snares of human understanding and reflection. And such an insight prescribes a certain course of action. The task that confronts us is not to liberate 'man' who languishes 'in the chains of external life', but rather to free him from 'an age-old load of false and distorted sincerity' which causes his words, gestures and movements to groan and falter (p. 6). The point is not to restore 'man' to his 'true (primitive)' place in an undivided world, but rather to tear down this very same dream, which is itself responsible for the entropy of 'the entire sphere of human expression':

> What could be more dishonest than to claim that words had somehow, at bottom, remained the same! I could not help seeing that the ashes of burnt-out meanings (and not only those) had covered what had, since time immemorial, been striving for expression in man's innermost soul. (p. 6)

One dream thus replaces another. (And one lie is recognized as another, the 'lies' that had been portrayed as profoundly inhabiting the world they described becoming instead just 'nasty lies the other side told me' (p. 7).) This other dream is one of other words and figures, other images and gestures, drawn from 'the remotest regions of the spirit' (p. 6). Not those which simply unveil themselves as an expression of 'truth' in the most simple, the most classical sense (truth as revelation). No, these words, figures, images, gestures are instead 'veiled and unveiled as in a dream' (p. 6) – as if in this *other* dream of the dream, an 'other' dream beneath the paintings of Edgar Jené:

When they meet in their heady course, and the spark of the wonderful is born from the marriage of strange and most strange, then I will know I am facing the new radiance. It will give me a dubious look because, even though I have conjured it up, it exists beyond the concepts of my wakeful thinking; its light is not daylight ... (p. 6).

The dream which unfolds within and against the supposed 'Kleistian' dream of the 'friend' (at the bottomless depths of the ocean or in the redoubling scenography of a puppet show) constitutes 'a new radiance'; a radiance which, nonetheless, casts a strange 'light' distinct from 'daylight'. Beyond 'the concepts of my waking thinking', it is a dream that reason cannot bring to the surface, which reason cannot face – although, for all that, it is a dream that remains lodged, immersed, within reason's dreams, the strange outcrop of its own visions. This dream distorts, dislocates: 'Its weight has a different heaviness; its colour speaks to the new eyes which my closed lids have given one another; my hearing has wandered into my fingertips and learns to see' (p. 6). Against – *right against* – the logos, a disseminating *différance* acquires a yet more original possibility.

Only then is Celan's text able to speak of (to dream of) the paintings of Edgar Jené, as if it were not just a matter of witnessing the surrealist transformation of the 'object' from the place where one 'is', but of experiencing a certain dislocation of the subject – that is, of one's own experience, one's own words and gestures – on the strength of a certain kind of dream, one that goes 'beneath' another dream (itself the product of 'waking thinking') which it cannot but resist and transform. The 'dangers' faced by 'tramping the deep sea ... following Edgar Jené down underneath his painting' thus occur at the point one in fact breaks off from listening 'to my own thoughts' (p. 7). If these 'dangers' are also the stakes of a certain 'freedom' (p. 7), as the text would have it, such 'freedom' cannot be thought of in terms of a pure return to an uncompromised 'self', since the self is, precisely, dislocated in the very cessation of thought, or transformation of thought, which takes us down beneath the dream.

Amid the sensory reconfiguration that sees colour speaking to new eyes, and hearing wandering into fingertips in order that it might learn to see, one cannot be sure just what one is 'seeing' in Edgar Jené's paintings (if it is even a matter of 'sight' in the simple sense). In *A Sail Leaves an Eye*, for instance, is there 'one sail only' or, in fact, 'two' (p. 7)? One of the two, if there are indeed two, perhaps does not leave – does that make the title of the painting more fitting? 'The first one, which still bears the colour of the eye, cannot proceed. I know it must come back' (p. 7). What leaves or journeys or 'sails' from the eye, if anything? And what, if anything, comes back? ('I know it must come back' is not the same as a return that has already occurred.) Is seeing a case of sight ventured, of which one can never be certain (does every 'sail' leave the eye)? Or is it a matter of sight returning vision to the eye ('I know it must come back') – the structure of which, if it is to remain operative, has a basic promissory form, thus *leaving* always the chance of a promise broken, an unfulfilled remainder? ('The first one will come home, into the empty, yet strangely seeing socket. Perhaps the tide will carry it in the wrong direction, into the eye which stares out on the grey of the other side … Then the boat will bear tidings, but without much promise.' (p. 7)). Or is the return all the more 'arduous', as the text puts it, for the fact that the 'first one … cannot proceed' at all? What does it mean for a 'sail' (that which supposedly sails from the eye) to *bear* the colour of an eye? Is it the picture that dramatizes these (unanswerable) questions? Or is it the dislocating 'experience' into which we must descend 'beneath Edgar Jené's paintings' that makes them possible? Does one properly come to Jené's paintings only after the 'dream about the dream' has paved the way? Or are the paintings already engulfed by it? In the confusion between what is seen of the painting, what is seen in it, and indeed whether and how it itself *sees*, the surrealist transformation – the dream '*about*' the dream – comes to pass. What – if anything – do we *see* of this, in a *text*? A text where 'my mouth, placed higher than my eyes and bolder for having often spoken in my sleep, had moved ahead and mocked me' (p. 4), yet also a text where 'colour speaks' – *speaks* – 'to the new eyes which my closed lids have given one another' (p. 6)?

The 'white profile' apparently visible in the painting constitutes a 'steep incline' which the sail 'climbs', climbing towards an 'eye without a pupil' – all that this profile 'owns' – as it journeys *with* rather than *against* the tide of an uphill flow of water (p. 7). The pupil-less eye, just because it is pupil-less, 'knows and can do more than we'. The profile (that of 'a woman with hair a little bluer than her mouth') looks up, 'diagonally, at a mirror we cannot see', as if testing her expression. She does not return our gaze (what, in any case, do we see?), and perhaps she does not return her own. The apparent interplay between the surreal spectacle of the painting, which does not remain within self-contained limits, and the surreal gaze of the viewer, which finds itself recast in the very image it contemplates, does not therefore give way to an identity or simple reciprocity, but is instead short-circuited precisely by the opacity of vision which in fact seems to connect the two (if two is, in any case, the right number here). If the profile is 'an icy monument at the access to the inner sea', the question of how to cross to the other side – 'What can the other side of this face look like?' – thus remains impossibly complicated. For it begs the question, from which 'side' do we see (if at all) that which 'sees', or which 'sees' us 'seeing' (if any), when we go beneath the paintings of Edgar Jené? From which 'side' does seeing come, if it comes at all? 'What can the other side of this face look like? – how would it look to us, or to itself? – or, how would it look itself? The crossing and the return of which the 'Kleistian' friend dreams is thus engulfed by this other dream, whereby 'the spark of the wonderful is born from the marriage of strange and most strange'. If 'then I will know I am facing the new radiance', nonetheless 'it will give me a dubious look' (p. 6).

The surrealist dream-journey (the dream *'about'* a dream) doesn't lead home, doesn't restitute (the) vision to itself, then, but instead takes us to the other side of vision itself, 'into the eye which stares out on the grey of the other side ...' (p. 7). 'We enter it in our sleep', says the text, 'then we see what remains to be dreamed' (p. 8).[3]

Sleep without Sleep

Compulsive pulsations: Survival, repetition and the *arrêt de mort*

As is well known, the double-banded text 'Living On/Borderlines'[1] was written for the 1979 collection *Deconstruction and Criticism*, which brought together essays by members of the Yale school – Harold Bloom, Paul de Man, Geoffrey Hartman, J. Hillis Miller, and Derrida himself – each of whom were asked by the publisher to write a new piece that took a specific literary example as the occasion to elucidate the main features of their own work. In reply, the contributors proposed Shelley's *The Triumph of Life* as a common literary source, although Derrida's own piece, in both its arguments and its textual performance, puts in question the very possibility of taking the poem as a core text or point of reference. The upper band of Derrida's contribution, 'Living On', explores the issue of the survival or living-on of literature. Here, Derrida grafts onto his reading of Shelley an exploration of two short texts by Maurice Blanchot, *La Folie du jour* (The Madness of the Day) and *L'Arrêt de mort* (Death Sentence) which for Derrida somehow translate the undecidability of Shelley's title, the double genitive of which implies both the triumph of life over death and death's triumphing over life. This very undecidability brings into view the problem of the 'literary' as a form of survival (a 'living-on' beyond the living-on of, say, a determinate author, or indeed a specific reader or reading), one that awaits decision in the face of the undecidable itself. 'Living On' may therefore be read alongside a host of other writings by Derrida including 'The Double Session', in which the *pharmakon* as undecidably both life-giving remedy and deathly poison is not to be considered a simple substance or essence but is instead characterized by an untranslatable self-difference at its origin.[2] Since it cannot, therefore, be reduced to a self-identical philosophical proposition or concept, but instead works its remedy/poison in the folds of philosophy's garments (indeed in the very lining of philosophy's self-enfoldedness), the *pharmakon* in effect provides one name for the problem of survival in the general – and always deconstructible – 'text' of the Western tradition.

Beneath 'Living On', meanwhile, the lower band, 'Borderlines', presents itself as an extended note to the translator of Derrida's writing. Here, Derrida poses questions concerning the possibility and limits of translation (his contribution was, in fact, earmarked for translation from the outset). Just as in writings such as 'Letter to a Japanese Friend',[3] this problem of translation is presented as inextricable for the very thinking of deconstruction. Institutional and disciplinary resistances to deconstruction's understanding of translatability are, for Derrida, bound up with this notion of the 'borderline', which is not only rethought but enacted quite differently at the always undecidable and divided limits of Derrida's double-banded text. For Derrida, the limits of translation are complicated from the beginning by the fact that the writing we might call 'literary' (itself far from a determinate field) may be read only in terms of a certain reference without referent. Thus, every text precisely *borders* on another, points towards or embarks upon another, yet in a way that ventures beyond those navigational tools and mooring techniques offered by a traditional conception of referentiality. (The original title of the piece, 'Journal de bord', translates more literally as shipboard journal.) This is perhaps just another way of speaking about living on, in the face of survival's own undecidable limits.

Living on as conquest of life in a double sense (life's triumph over death in the very form of its survival, but also death's constitutive importance in defining that survival itself as a modality of life) is, as Derrida tells us, best described as a 'reprieve' or an 'afterlife', '"life after life" or life after death, more life or more than life, and better, the state of suspension in which it's over – *and* over again, and you'll have never have done with that suspension itself' (p. 77). The aporia of living on as at once death sentence and suspension of death gives rise to an absolutely impassable situation which is nonetheless never tranquil or static, but always characterized by a restless and irresolvable repeatability. Indeed, the very problem of this aporetic situation is itself compounded and perhaps engulfed by the impossibility of its description *as such*. For, as Derrida himself asks in 'Living On': 'Who is … little enough alive, or alive enough, to dare speak about living?' (p. 78). If the critical distance or detachment needed to properly isolate 'life' as an object of knowledge in the classical sense would put philosophical inquiry in the very grip of death, equally the affinity that is effectively required to identify the very same 'object' as an object *for us* would imbue the inquirer with more 'life' than mere disinterestedness would allow. How could one not participate in the object of one's interest, where that object is 'life' itself? But, then again, on the strength of this very same (critical) *interest*, how could one ever participate in it fully or *as such*? The problem of the *arrêt de mort* as the suspension of life-death is, then, not simply to be stated; instead, it everywhere performs itself, precisely in terms of the impossible situation that the question of the *arrêt de mort* brings about. (As Derrida says of *L'Arrêt de mort*, albeit in slightly different circumstances, 'the narrative is the very event that it recounts' (p. 145).)

The verb *arrêter* that in Derrida's reading organizes Blanchot's text (though not without disorganizing its hermeneutic availability as such) doesn't just act as a pivotal point. Rather, it 'twice marks the boundary that brings things to an end only to let them start and start over or start on again' (p. 112). Thus:

> The *arrêt de mort* is not only the decision that determines what cannot be decided: it also arrests death by suspending it, interrupting it, deferring with a "start" {*sursaut*} the startling starting over, and starting on, of living on. But then what suspends or holds back death is the very thing that gives it its undecidability – another false name, rather than pseudonym, for differance. (p. 114)

This repeatability of the *arrêt de mort*, precisely due to the intensity of its aporetic irresolution, can no more be grouped into a knowable sequence or predictable pattern than it can be reduced to a simplistic notion of the 'pure' or unique event – a simple 'one-off' – unmarked by the trace structure of writing in the general sense. Rather, each 'start' – each 'arrhythmic pulsation of its syntax' (p. 114) – marks upon the 'here-and-now' the event of a radically unknowable 'to come' which nevertheless structures and de-structures its very possibility. Indeed, death in its constitutive suspension is also tied by Derrida to a certain 'dissemination of the rhythm of life with no finishing stroke' (p. 121): the ending to life, which might perhaps grant its telos, would nevertheless be akin to what Agamben terms the end of the poem as it falls into prose and thus non-poetry,[4] thus making the end itself *improper*, rather than simply an end-in-itself or of-itself. The finishing stroke would therefore be a stroke no longer, no longer a syntactic 'pulsation'. There would be, then, no possibility of a 'finishing stroke', and this would define the event of the *arrêt de mort* as much as its originary divisibility.

Here, we might cross the border to another text by Derrida, 'Shibboleth', which he writes on Paul Celan.[5] For Derrida, Celan's texts constitute extraordinary literary events to the extent that they are at once irreplaceably singular acts of writing and testaments to the always repeatable and divisible trait of every singularity. This means that, even in its absolute and untranslatable uniqueness, a poem inscribes itself – here and now, for one time only – in conditions and contexts which nevertheless permit, indeed demand, that it be read or re-read and repeated. The poem in its most original marking (or its marked originality) is thus, from the outset, given to be re-marked, transcribed, translated in some way. That Celan's poetry performs this paradox with such acuity cannot be wholly disentangled from the events of the poet's own life and history, since his poems' intensely singular qualities are both threatened and heightened at every turn by the risk they always run of being, as Derrida himself puts it, 'exported, deported, expropriated, reappropriated' (p. 6).

In 'Shibboleth', the repeatability that always accompanies the possibility of a singular incision in writing here comes down to a question of what we might call the 'date'. Like the signature and the proper name, the date incisively marks that which is irreplaceable or unsubstitutable. Yet the date is also given to be repeated or re-marked as the very condition of its possibility. Thus, dating calls for a certain readability or return at another time and in another place. From the very beginning, then, the date carries away the text that it nevertheless marks as irreplaceably singular, impelling it towards an other (other-of-itself) yet to come, rather than simply tying it to a past that may be determined or objectified as such. And for Derrida all texts worthy of their name are in some way signed/dated – as particular and remarkable openings in language and history – just as all readings and re-markings are in some way dated/signed. Hence, once it is written, the text we are given to read is not simply abandoned to some universal possibility or expansive generality for all time to come, but instead returns to be read *on another day*. Indeed, that every reading comes down to a re-marked date implies that reading is itself an act or event of commemoration, the coming to pass of something like an anniversary. Once more, that the reading of his poetry brings out such issues for Derrida cannot be wholly extricated from the fact that Celan writes as survivor. He writes, indeed, as one who not only preserves and commemorates dates (not least, those of a certain twentieth-century Europe), but who insists – as part of precisely the same gesture – that they exceed (i.e. survive) both the objectifications of history – including the dry observation or commemoration of anniversaries – and the grasp of philosophical mastery.

To say that the poetic text in its singular repeatability – its *datedness* – crosses from one time (and, inevitably, one place) to another, is to suggest that such traversal of borders is imperative for acts of poetry to take place. Such crossing, in other words, is poetry's very condition. (Here, one thinks of Derrida's 'Che cosè la poesia',[6] in which the poem is thought of as a hedgehog that self-protectively balls itself up in the middle of the road, bristling its spines at the traffic that may traverse its crossing and indeed threaten its existence, although of course in just this situation its existence must nevertheless be ventured.) Hence, the poem comes to define itself not in terms of a 'content' that might be reproduced intact, as the 'object' of a knowledge; instead, poetry enacts itself performatively, in the very experience or event of a crossing which cannot be reduced to such a self-same 'object'. Thus it is that Derrida comes to dwell on a Hebrew word found in one of Celan's poems: shibboleth. Shibboleth is a password that must be given at the border, becoming the very test of passage across. As Derrida observes, the Ephraimites knew the password but could not pronounce it correctly, saying 'sibboleth' instead. It was this that betrayed them – not a lack of knowledge, but of performative ability. And since the shibboleth comes down to more than just an inert repetition of the self-same, Derrida tells us that it multiplies at the borders, cropping up in a host of languages: Phoenician, Judeo-Aramaic, Syriac. In a sense, shibboleth belongs nowhere but at the border (a borderline of survivors, as all borderlines surely are). As a password, it is a cipher that does not harbour any essential meaning, and thus gathers within itself only the possibility and commemoration of innumerable migra-tions. It is itself multiply crossed. Rather than returning to memory some elemental and indivisible 'truth' or ground, it re-enacts and re-encrypts that non-signifying difference (*différance*) which traverses the very body of the mark. Thus, the poem as shibboleth speaks beyond knowledge.

The shibboleth, in other words, commemorates the borders of life-death, producing a still-inventable 'truth' of those borders, rather than a knowledge of them as such. The temporality – or, rather, the 'arrythmic pulsation' – of the *arrêt de mort* would seem to correspond in certain respects to this multiply crossed code-word whose 'meaning' always remains to come, remaining in abeyance, even and especially as it performs itself in the 'here and now'. Shibboleth, *l'arrêt de mort*: something happens, will have happened, again, we can't know it for sure, on the very borderlines of survival.

Derrida writes of the *arrêt*, 'No consciousness, no perception, no watchfulness can gather up this remnance, this *restance*; no attentiveness can make it present, no "I", no ego; hence its essential relationship to ghosts, fantasies, daydreams, to *Phantasieren* (Freud) or the "waking dream" (*The Triumph of Life*)'. That which 'retains the title and assures the compulsive pulsation of *L'Arrêt de mort*' amounts to an 'epochal [etym. epokhe, "pause"; in phenomenology, "bracketing"] suspension' (p. 116).

Sleep, suspension

How, in *L'Arrêt de mort*,[7] does this 'epochal suspension' manifest itself, as that which compulsively pulsates so as to conjure a certain spectrality beyond all consciousness, perception, or ordinary attentiveness? Permit me to quote a lengthy passage which Blanchot gives us to read, just a few pages after the rather more dramatic 'return to life' that follows the entire scenography of J.'s apparent death:

> … I closed the door. At that moment she really dozed off, into an almost calm sleep, and I was watching her live and sleep when all of a sudden she said with great anguish "Quick, a perfect rose," all the while continuing to sleep but now with a slight rattle. The nurse came and whispered to me that the night before that word had been the last she had pronounced: when she had seemed to be sunk in complete unconsciousness, she had abruptly awakened from her stupor to point to the oxygen balloon and murmur, "A perfect rose," and had immediately sunk again.

This story chilled me. I told myself that what had happened the night before, from which I had been excluded, was beginning all over again ... I took her hand gently, by the wrist (she was sleeping), and scarcely had I touched it when she sat up with her eyes open, looked at me furiously and pushed me away, saying, "Never touch me again." Then immediately she stretched out her arms to me, just as in the morning, and burst into tears. She cried, she sobbed against me in such a transport of grief that she was on the point of suffocating ...

She fell asleep again. Her sleep had a strange way of dissolving in an instant, so that behind it she seemed to remain awake and be grappling with serious matters there, in which I played perhaps a terrifying role. She had fallen asleep, her face wet with tears. Far from being spoiled by it, her youth seemed dazzling ... A little later, however, her expression changed. Almost under my eyes, the tears had dried and the tear stains had disappeared; she became severe, and her slightly raised lips showed the contraction of her jaw and her tightly clenched teeth, and gave her a rather mean and suspicious look; her hand moved in mine to free itself, I wanted to release it, but she seized me again right away with a savage quickness in which there was nothing human. When the nurse came to me – in a low voice and about nothing important – J. immediately awoke and said in a cold way, "I have my secrets with her too." She went back to sleep at once. (pp. 25–6)

This scene does more than merely depict the near-death delirium of J., semi-sedated (and yet equally unsettled, as she undoubtedly is) by the administering of oxygen and painkilling drugs. It does more, too, than stage the ambivalent and unstable projections of the narrator, whose attempts to write himself into this almost unwitnessable drama – sometimes with a near parodic degree of narcissism – are continually stymied by the whole series of impenetrable suspensions encountered here, between life and death, wakefulness and sleep (throughout the text, sleep and insomnia aren't stably distinguished – as if sleep was always already inhabited by its own refusal, by insomnia itself), epiphanies and secrets, allegory and bare truth, touch and its prohibition, control and loss of control, the human and the inhuman, meaning and non-meaning. If, as Derrida contends, 'the narrative is the very event that it recounts', in this passage we find that the very possibility of narration – of narrativity itself – draws close to its own suspension (though never to a simple 'ending'). Meanwhile, on the borderlines of just these suspensive states, sleep recurs, returns. For sure, it is not 'natural' sleep, 'normal', healthy repose, the kind of sleep that happens according to the regular rhythms of everyday life, coming in controlled doses in order to support the demands of common-place daytime existence. (Throughout *L'Arrêt de mort* one is not gently lulled to sleep, nor does one awake comfortably, slowly; instead, sleep starts and stops suddenly, quickly, with hardly a delay, if it happens at all – it comes and goes with a rapidity that at once alienates and pervades 'life' in the ordinary sense.) But, let's pause for a moment – just this description of 'natural' sleep as controlled, regulated activity suggests it is much more like the drug-induced state of J. than we might otherwise think. Thus, sleep is in fact less of a natural occurrence untouched by human endeavour than a highly determined and constructed phenomenon, produced and managed in very specific ways to serve the interests of the 'day'. Sleep, in other words, is not so much 'natural' as it is *naturalized*. In this scene from *L'Arrêt de mort*, then, repeated reference to the oxygen balloon works not so much to contrast J.'s drug-addled slip-sliding toward unconsciousness with the onset of 'natural' sleep, as to overwrite the distinction between the two, giving us instead an unsettling and highly ambivalent image of sleep on the borderline of a whole series of suspensive states – a 'sleep' which at once produces and limits the possibility of 'consciousness' or 'perception' in all their (constructible) effects. This 'sleep' – crossed as it is with delirium, daydreaming, and the distorted poetry of the 'perfect rose', touched madly by a love-hate touching (a 'touch', that is, which may be both stroke and strike), bordering on a vigilance beyond all possible vigilance – this 'sleep' is nothing other than the suspensive medium of life-death. It is on its border-lines that the 'arrythmic pulsation' of the *arrêt de mort* happens as impossible event – 'the state of suspension in which it's over – *and* over again, and you'll never have done with that suspension itself'.

And yet Derrida's 'Living On' makes nothing of sleep. Amid the complex disseminal play which underscores the trace structure of survival itself, 'sleep' is sidelined according to a gesture which, though unstated, draws perilously close to the more crudely physiological understanding of slumber that one may detect in philosophy or critical thought from a certain Aristotle onwards. Sleep does not feature in the disseminal chain of non-substitutable terms – *différance*, trace, supplement, cinder, shibboleth, pharmakon, living-on – which, in turn, excludes it only at the risk of implying sleep's self-evident naturality. In this rather complex sense, sleep emerges, perhaps, as the (unavowed) condition of living on.

'The dream of a dream that comes to an end', 'the movement of looking into oneself'

In his essay, 'Dreaming, Writing',[8] Blanchot considers the dreams of Michel Leiris, recounted in his *Nuits sans nuit et quelques jours sans jour*. In one dream, Leiris imagines himself looking through an opening above a darkened enclosure, only to find that he is looking into himself. For Blanchot, this anguished dream is not 'provoked by the discovery of the strange realities contained in one's inner depths'. Rather, it characterizes only 'the movement of looking into oneself, where there is nothing to see but the constriction of a closed space without light'. Several years later, another dream of Leiris's 'reconsiders this movement', as Blanchot puts it. It is 'the dream of a dream that comes to an end, but instead of ascending to an awakening in an effort to rise and to emerge, this dream surreptitiously invites the dreamer to find an exit from below, that is, to enter into the depths of another sleep that will no doubt never end' (p. 141). For Blanchot a strange economy links, on the one hand, the abyssal dream-scene that sees the gaze move towards the impossible spectacle of its 'self' (itself), and, on the other, an interminable vigilance beyond vigilance found in the very deep of sleep, a vigilance which operates at the most radical limit of dreaming construed as an extension of consciousness, no matter how complex this extension may be:

> What these two dreams have in common, what is grasped and lived as image by both of them, is the very movement of turning back: in the first dream, a turning back upon oneself such that simple imagery might attribute it to introspection; in the second, a turning back of the dream as if it were turning back to surprise or watch over itself, identifying thus, with an inverse vigilance, a state of wakefulness of the second degree in search of its own limit. (p. 141)

The dream of dreaming's end, which leads not to an awakening to the 'day' but instead to a deeper descent into another sleep – a sleep beyond dreams – seems to invite the interminable, the boundless, the 'without end' (in at least a multiple sense). This is a sleep, in other words, that is at once beyond-death and not-death: *l'arrêt de mort*. Such a dreamless sleep therefore conjures the *arrêt* of which Derrida speaks: 'No consciousness, no perception, no watchfulness can gather up this remnance, this *restance*; no attentiveness can make it present, no "I", no ego …'. And yet this abyssal 'turning back of the dream' upon itself happens *as if* the impossible spectacle of a gaze's movement towards the vision of its 'self'/itself were simply being replayed otherwise. As if the hyper-vigilance – the vigilance beyond all possible vigilance – that this extraordinary scene implies recurs at or *as* the most radical limit of dreaming, 'identifying it thus', endlessly watching over its impossible quest for self-identification.

Within the space of a few lines, Blanchot is quick to distinguish the dreamer from the sleeper. 'The one who dreams turns away from the one who sleeps; the dreamer is not the sleeper' (p. 141). Frequently the dream contrives the sense that one is not dreaming, and therefore not asleep. Even when one's dream conveys the sense that one is indeed dreaming, this 'flight into a more inner dream' is nonetheless accompanied by an awareness of the dream taking place, which provokes 'an endless flight outside the dream' (p. 141), or in other words a certain turning back towards wakefulness even as the dream becomes increasingly self-reflexive or all-engulfing. In both these cases, then, the dream seemingly cannot help but recreate some sense of waking life (thus turning the dream away from sleep). And yet, Blanchot asks: 'In the dream, who is dreaming? Who is the "I" of the dream? Who is the person to whom one attributes this "I," admitting that there is one?' Blanchot's own response to this question is a complex one:

> Between the one who sleeps and the one who is the subject of the dream's plot, there is a fissure, the hint of an interval and a difference of structure; of course it is not truly another, another person, but what is it? (p. 141)

Now, the obvious thing to say about this remark is that Blanchot well appreciates that the 'I' which emerges and is experienced in dreams is, precisely, 'the subject of the dream's plot' – a figure and function of the narrative or structure of the dream – rather than a simple expression of the personhood of somebody who exists in waking life. This waking 'I' could, of course, be similarly construed as itself a fictional projection, a condition of a whole series of discourses, etc., but the point here is that each operates in a distinct economy, so that either one may not simply be overlaid upon the other. Nonetheless, Blanchot does not insist upon an absolute non-relation between the two, but rather 'a difference of structure', 'the hint of an interval', or 'a fissure' which precisely constitutes their relation ('of course it is not truly another, another person ...'). Upon awakening, Blanchot observes, we often 'greedily take possession of the night's adventures, as if they belonged to us', though with a seemingly unavoidable feeling both of 'usurpation' and 'gratitude' (pp. 141–2). In other words, the very disposition of the 'self' is produced precisely by this 'interval' or 'fissure' which permits the self to enter into a movement towards itself. The 'I' is constituted in all its effects by this movement towards itself as if it were another, or, better still, by this movement towards the other of itself as if it were the 'self' itself.[9] 'Usurpation' and 'gratitude', when put together, imply nothing less than the sovereign gift of the 'I'-to-itself. Yet this situation is possible only on the strength of a structuring difference for which the dream itself stands. Neither the 'I' in the dream nor the 'I' of waking life constitute an authentic, self-identical or even predominating 'self'; rather, the sovereign gift of the 'I'-to-itself depends upon just this 'interval' or 'fissure' which, precisely, gives the 'I' to itself (though not without the intractable remainder of 'intrigue', of an 'irreducible distance' which is also a distance-without-distance of sorts (p. 142), presumably one that would engender a sense of self-doubt, alienation or even shame as much as complacent self-regard, as indeed Blanchot suggests when he says that 'we are in the position of strangers in the dream ... because the I of the dreamer does not have the meaning of a real I' (p. 144)). Almost by definition, this structuring difference – from which one cannot take a reliable distance – is no more recuperable than it can be dispensed with. The 'distance between me and myself' (p. 142) cannot be reclaimed by the 'I' it makes possible. It cannot be experienced as a feature of the 'I' for which it is nonetheless a precondition. In other words, it is that which 'watches over' the *dream* of wakefulness itself, a wakefulness 'always in search of its own limit' (p. 141), always seeking itself at its own borders. 'No consciousness, no perception, no watchfulness can gather up this remnance, this *restance*; no attentiveness can make it present, no "I", no ego ...'. 'It' 'watches', vigilant beyond viligance, at the limit of dreams.

At the most remote edge of dreaming, therefore, one perhaps finds a sort of originary anonymity which awaits us, a near abyssal other that remains nonetheless (at) the supplementing limit of every subject. The dream makes of us a 'stranger' to ourselves, since the dream reveals itself 'to someone who is not there in person and does not have the status of a subject who is present':

> One could even say that there is no one in the dream and therefore, in some
> sense, no one to dream it; whence the suspicion that when we are dreaming, it is
> just as easily someone else who is dreaming and who dreams us, someone who
> in turn, in dreaming us, is being dreamed by someone else, a premonition of the
> dream without dreamer, which would be the dream of the night itself. (p. 144)

Being dreamt by another, by someone else in turn dreamt by some other who
in the end cannot even be figured as 'dreamer' – this is 'the dream of the night
itself' (p. 144). The dream draws us close to literature, perhaps, not on the
strength of its capacity to convey autobiographical or psychoanalytic 'truth', but
through an 'exactness of relation' whereby the dream offers the possibility of a
'literary affirmation' of those 'poetic signs' which make up dreams themselves,
while also confronting them with their own 'exteriority' in the sense that
writing and the dream do not ever simply coincide as co-present events (pp.
142–3). (This non-coincidence in fact not only determines the relationship of
writing to dreaming, but presumably also structures the self-difference, the
spectrality, of each.) Without simple origin in an existential, autobiographical
or psychical 'self', dreams throw up resemblances without end – images of
friends, for instance, whereby 'each person tends to be extremely, marvelously
resemblant'. 'A being who suddenly begins to "resemble" moves away from
real life', Blanchot tells us, 'passes into another world, enters the inaccessible
proximity of the image, is present nonetheless, with a presence that is not his
own or that of another, an apparition that transforms all other presents into
appearances' (p. 145). The dream thus gives us pure images, pure image itself,
resemblances whose structuring principle dispenses with the logic of both the
representation of the 'object' and of the 'subject'. Reference without ultimate
referent; thus, always already, and everywhere, at each border (without ultimate
border), an 'inaccessible proximity' of the image. Here, as we shall see, it is the
corpse that offers Blanchot a prime image of this image, since it reveals itself in
terms of a resemblance no longer grounded in an existent thing. (Let us note
for the time being, however, that the corpse is a 'strange, beautiful being who is
like his double slowly resurfacing from the depths' (p. 145).) Thus, the dream is
'the place of similitude, an environment saturated with resemblances where a
neutral power of resembling, which exists prior to any particular designation, is
ceaselessly in search of some figure that it elicits, if need be, in order to settle on
it' (p. 145). We, dreamers, are figured by this movement of resemblance which

itself exceeds – as much as it makes possible – the logic of the figure. It is in this sense, perhaps, that Blanchot wants to say that 'the dream is a temptation for writing' (p. 147). Writing longs for the 'neutral vigilance' that is attemptedly extinguished by 'the night of sleep' – sleep in the ordinary sense, that is, sleep construed in time-honoured fashion as merely the temporary deprivation of sense-perception brought about to serve the utile interests of the 'day'. This 'neutral vigilance' is awakened, instead, by the 'night of dream' – a night bathed in the shadowless light or impenetrable darkness of an empty image, the 'nothing to see' which, in looking back at us, resembles us. Writing, needless to say, dreams of nothing other than 'imitating this power to imitate and to resemble that is without origin' (p. 147). Such a dream, however, is 'the dream of the night itself', at the most radical limit of the dreamer. It is the very 'deep of sleep' construed as a 'refusal to sleep at the heart of sleep' – construed, that is, not in terms of the perpetual psychic restlessness which supposedly provokes dreaming as the expression of an ever-sensate cerebrum incapable of peaceful slumber, but rather in terms of a ceaseless movement of difference and resemblance without origin which goes beyond and before the very possibility of the subject who, we suppose, 'dreams'. Thus, while the 'insomnia' that Blanchot repeatedly valorizes as the inspiration for writing is indeed placed in stark contrast to a 'night of sleep' in the ordinary sense, its very character nonetheless partakes of that which falls from sleep in sleep, that which takes the dream to the very limit of itself, and which indeed dreams its end without end.

In a short text for Robert Antelme, 'In the Night That is Watched Over',[10] Blanchot begins: 'It is slowly, in those nights when I sleep without sleeping, that I became conscious (this word is inappropriate) of your proximity, which is distant nonetheless' (p. 133). And, from *The Writing of the Distaster*[11]: 'The writer, daytime insomniac' (p. 121); 'Kafka … knows that writing is madness already, his madness, a kind of vigilance, unrelated to any wakefulness save sleep's: insomnia' (p. 43).

'What there is in the deep of sleep'

In 'Sleep, Night' (a short text included in *The Space of Literature*),[12] during a paragraph we shall have cause to come back to, Blanchot writes:

> By means of sleep, day uses night to block out the night. Sleep belongs to the world: it is a task. We sleep in accord with the general law which makes our daytime activity depend on our nightly repose ... far from being a dangerous, bewitching force, sleep will become domesticated and serve as the instrument of our power to act. We surrender to sleep, but in the way that the master entrusts himself to the slave who serves him. Sleeping is the clear action which promises us to the day ... Only deep sleep lets us escape what there is in the deep of sleep. (p. 264)

Blanchot scorns sleep in its more conventional conception as merely instrumental to the needs of the day, Here, he reprises Kant's – and, for that matter, Hegel's – image of the somnambulist as a troubling figure, although the lack of explicit reference to either Kant or Hegel may itself imply that philosophy, an ostensibly 'honest profession', is in fact something of a shady business, conducted under cover of darkness:

> Nocturnal wandering, the tendency to stray when the world is attenuated and grows distant, and even the honest professions which are necessarily practised at night attract suspicions. To sleep with open eyes is an anomaly symbolically indicating something which the general consciousness does not approve of. People who sleep badly always appear more or less guilty. What do they do? They make night present. (p. 265)

Thus, sleep as the rational instrument of waking life represses the very 'deep of sleep' which nevertheless dwells at the 'other' origin of (its) night. The sleeper who represses this 'other night' can say 'I sleep', but this self-assured evocation of a sovereign 'masterable-possible' implies a paradoxical state of affairs, since sleep thereby becomes merely the mirror-image of the day, a simple reflection of day-time interests and concerns. (Somnabulism makes troublingly visible this irreducible crossing of sleep with non-sleep.) The sleeper's attentiveness to the day – in the form of day-oriented night-time dreams – may nevertheless pose a radical threat to the day itself. 'Whoever does not sleep cannot stay awake', writes Blanchot (p. 265). This enigmatic maxim resonates, as we shall see, with some of Levinas's writings of around the same period, in which sleep is seen as a precondition for consciousness as a particular form of being. But it might also point to a deep tension in the normative relation of 'night' to 'day', waking to sleeping. For the 'sleeplessness' of ordinary sleep – its functional orientation towards the interests of the day – implies continuous and continual day in effect, and thus in effect a *non-day*, a day which cannot differentiate itself as such. This would be a day *as* non-day to which the slumberer of the 'night of sleep' might therefore never awaken.

The dream of instrumental – that is, day-oriented – sleep is characterized by Blanchot in the following way (we shall see that this passage is much indebted to Levinas):

> I retire from the world's immensity and its disquietude, but in order to give myself to the world, which is maintained, thanks to my "attachment," in the sure truth of a limited and circumscribed place. Sleep is my absolute interest in assuring myself of the world. From this limit which sleep provides, I take hold of the world by its finite side: I grasp it firmly enough so that it stays, puts me in place, puts me to rest. To sleep badly is precisely to be unable to find one's position. (p. 265)

Seeming withdrawal from the world during night-time remakes the very possibility of a reawakening to the world and to oneself in the world ('absolute interest'), allowing the self to remake itself in the world and remake the world for itself ('to find one's position'). This idea of sleep recalls Kant's notion of slumber as 'a relaxation, which is nevertheless at the same time a gathering of power for renewed external sensations'. Yet, to reprise a theme of Blanchot's once more, 'Sleep, Night' suggests that within the heart of sleep – in another sleep beyond sleep – there is also a certain vigilance which must more radically interrupt itself, exceed itself, or enter into the abyss of itself. In one sense, vigilance would not seem to be suspended by means of the ordinary sleep which, since it serves waking life, turns out to be no deeper sleep at all, but only the observance of 'day' in another guise. On the other hand, however, vigilance oriented towards the day is, more radically, nothing but the absence of vigilance itself (it is, in other words, a drowsy servitude). Hence, it is by recourse to a vigilance that is 'other' than ordinary vigilance that radical or absolute vigilance persists, as something like a remainder or excess at the heart of vigilance, which is at once constitutive of and irrecuperable to vigilance itself. As Herschel Farbman puts it, in his book *The Other Night*, what awakens as the sleeper sleeps is, in Blanchot, something like a 'neutral vigilance that continues, in sleep, where the subject leaves off' (p. 51). 'Neutral', to be understood in terms of a certain 'intrusion of the other', as Blanchot says in *The Infinite Conversation*.[13] Thus an 'other night' inhabits the night of sleep, ruining restful slumber in a more profound way than by mere negation of sleep. Ruining 'simple' sleep, in other words, by grounding its dream of vigilance – for instance, the Kantian dream of near-drowning which awakens the sleeper and prevents their death – in an 'other' which persists at the very heart of what sleep and dreaming come to awaken as possibility.

This 'other' night, then, is a night within-sleep-beyond-sleep. In 'Sleep, Night', Blanchot writes: 'Night, the essence of night, does not let us sleep. In the night no refuge is to be found in sleep … In the night one cannot sleep' (pp. 266–7). For Blanchot, as we have seen, to sleep in the ordinary sense is to do nothing more than prepare for and thus serve the day – a day construed by the world as decisively 'non-night'. If 'night' is therefore in essence at odds with sleep in its functional sense, the dream brings us closer to the 'nocturnal region' (p. 267), says Blanchot – although this is not at all the same as Kant's childhood dream of near-drowning, which merely saves the day. Indeed, Blanchot remarks that such a day is in fact not what the world thinks; it is, rather, 'the approach of time's absence, the threat of the outside where the world lacks' (p. 267). Ordinary sleep seeks at once to reassert and repress the truth of this interminable or 'timeless' day, to preserve its ceaseless dominion while at the same time upholding the impression of its temporal (i.e. world-making) reinscription and elevation (over night) as 'day'. The dream, then, is for Blanchot nothing other than 'the reawakening of the interminable' in the form of 'the approach of time's absence' which sleep cannot fully repress, since sleep is also its servant (p. 267). The 'interminable' is, therefore, less a sign of the day's power over nightfall, than it is the threat of a certain irrecuperable yet constitutive 'outside' (i.e. the absent time or non-time beyond the day that nonetheless defines the dominion or sovereignty of the day, at once constituting and threatening its 'presence' from the perspective of a double or redoubling 'lack'). This dream – the 'reawakening of the interminable' – is thus a sleep-resisting core that lodges in the very breast of sleep as a consequence of day's radical deconstructibility carried over into night.[14] It is a dream that, in a sense, sleep's impossibility *as such* makes possible.

The interminable 'outside' ('the threat of the outside where the world lacks', 'the approach of time's absence') which makes and unmakes the sleeper's dream can't simply be returned to the day to which it nevertheless seems to belong. Yet, as Blanchot remarks elsewhere in *The Space of Literature*, 'to write is to surrender to the fascination of time's absence' (p. 30), as if whatever we find in the impossible space of the dream is also at the beginning of writing itself. To write: Blanchot speaks of nearing the 'essence of solitude' here, a 'solitude' which constitutes itself – against the perfectly closed intimacy of the self with itself that one impossibly seeks in the soundest sleep or the purest rest – through the bursting forth of an exposure to the outside which dreams continually bring. Thus, in *The Space of Literature*, the night of writing beckons to one who is nonetheless *not* destined to fulfil a vocation (i.e. to master the other), since its 'fascination' has – or, rather, *gives* – 'no power, it does not call, it attracts only by negligence':

> Whoever believes he is attracted finds himself profoundly neglected. Whoever claims to be in the thrall of an irresistible vocation, is only dominated by his own weakness. He calls irresistible the fact that there is nothing to resist; he calls vocation that which does not call him, and he has to shoulder his nothingness for a yoke. (p. 170)

Inspiration for Blanchot is therefore quashed, rather than embraced or endured, by those who seek to immerse themselves in night as an expression of the writerly vocation (a vocation of undoubtedly worldly benefit, bringing as it does honours and accomplishments). Such an approach at once denies and deepens the 'void' (the fissuring relation?) to which the other night exposes us beyond ourselves. Instead, it is the impossibility of the work that is suffered in the very experience of the night, which cannot be confronted head-on, nor put to a stop ('there is no exact moment at which one could pass from night to the *other* night, no limit at which to stop and come back in the other direction' (p. 169)). Hence, for Blanchot, writing 'begins with Orpheus's gaze' (p. 176), and therefore with the impossibility of reducing experience to an object of perception or the production of a work which finds its origin in the subject (or which takes its meaning to be the redemption of the subject).

For Farbman, then, the endless *mis en abyme* which characterizes the dream does not lead the dreamer into pure narcissistic self-enclosure, but on the contrary exposes them to 'the outside which has no location and affords no rest', as *The Space of Literature* has it (p. 31). This is also the 'region' where, as Blanchot tells us, 'pure resemblance reigns' to the extent that there is, in Farbman's terms, no 'original model', no 'initial revelation', no 'point of departure' to anchor dreams securely. Thus, in 'Sleep, Night', the dream is pure image – a 'likeness that refers eternally to likeness' (p. 268). It constitutes a resemblance that ultimately has nothing to resemble – or, in other words, a structure of experience without simple recourse to, as Farbman himself puts it, 'the logic of the representation of objects' (p. 62). Farbman shows how, in Blanchot, the corpse provides the very image of this image, since, as we have seen, it offers a resemblance no longer grounded in an existent thing. Yet, as Farbman writes, the 'corpse is not only an image of an absent person ... but also an image of the absence of the object' (p. 61). Indeed, since the irreducible possibility of the object's absence in general provides the conditions for the idea of a corpse in particular, for Farbman the corpse is just 'the image of a corpse, which is to say the image of an image ad infinitum'. As 'objectless image of itself and thus as errant movement' utterly beyond repose, the corpse, he argues, has a telling relation to writing as 'the movement of image as image' (p. 62). Here, he cites *The Space of Literature* once more:

> In literature, doesn't language itself become altogether image? We do not mean a language containing images or one that casts reality in figures, but one that is its own image ... a language, that is, which issues from its own absence, the way the image emerges upon the absence of the thing; a language addressing itself to the shadow of events as well, not to their reality ... and this because of the fact that the words that express them are not signs but images, images of words, and words where things turn into images. (Cited in Farbman, p. 34)

Literature is thus the image of language not in the sense of being the literary representation of a prior object (i.e. the linguistic field as, in turn, a representational tool oriented by a given reality). Instead, literature gives language *as* image 'in the same way as the corpse is the image of itself', says Farbman (p. 63) – indeed in just the same way that the corpse is the image of an image. The question of literature in Blanchot, Farbman argues, is therefore nothing less than the 'general problem of the restlessness of the corpse – the restlessness of the image as image even, and especially, in the very image of final rest' (p. 64). The corpse, like the sleeping body, provides only an *image* of rest yet must be thought of according to a logic of the image itself, which brooks no essential repose. Yet whether we are talking about writing 'as the movement of image as image', or the dream as radical exposure to the other beyond the mastery or sovereignty of the 'I', the restlessness found at the origin of literature cannot be thought in terms of a dialecticizable opposition to sleep, precisely to the extent that such restlessness entails the impossible 'experience' of a radical absencing of the subject – something like the death which, as *The Space of Literature* says of the experience of writing, 'happens to no one' (p. 33),[15] thus emerging only as if it were dreamt (beyond the dreamer), only ever as image, image of image. If, as Farbman argues, 'disaster' for Blanchot 'names the impossibility of resting in sleep, and even in death', the restless movement of dreaming or writing – beyond the stable moorings of both 'subject' and 'object' – depends on a falling away of the subject, a falling away which falls to the fall (rather than the fullness) of sleep. Blanchot's writing exposes the sleep of reason which occurs in the very promise of perfect day, a promise which mutates in the dream he associates with the 'other night', a dream which harbours the irrepressible return of 'time's absence', and which opens on to the very 'outside' which the world – and the self – lacks or *wants* (as much as 'world' or 'self' seek to overcome this 'outside' as such). As Blanchot writes, 'only deep sleep' – the sound night-time slumber of the man of action – lets us escape 'what there is in the deep of sleep'.

'The reawakening of the *there is* in the heart of negation'

For Levinas, writing in the late 1940s, 'the irremissibility of pure existing', as he puts it in *Time and the Other*,[16] is to be thought of in terms of the anonymous vigilance of the *'there is'* (*il y a*). The sheer fact of the *'there is'* remains radically prior or excessive in regard to any form of existent being. Even should there no longer be anything, pure existing implacably returns in absolutely impersonal form. ('It is impersonal like "it is raining" or "it is hot"', Levinas tells us (p. 47).) Beyond the polarities of negation and affirmation, the *'there is'* irrecuperably persists:

> This existing cannot be purely and simply affirmed, because one always affirms a *being* [*étant*]. But it imposes itself because one cannot deny it. Behind every negation this ambience of being, this being as a "field of forces" reappears, as the field of every affirmation and negation. It is never attached to an object *that is*, and because of this I call it anonymous. (p. 47)

Levinas wants to think of this irremissible pure existing, over and above all existent beings, in terms of insomnia. 'Insomnia', he writes, 'is constituted by the consciousness that it will never finish, that is, that there is no longer any way of withdrawing from the vigilance to which one is held. Vigilance without end.' For Levinas, insomnia shares with pure existing the sheer impossibility

of interruption or intermission. It remains closed to the possibility of unconsciousness. It is forever blocked from consoling retreat into a demarcated
interiority. The '*there is*' must therefore be thought of in terms of an utter
vigilance 'without possible recourse to sleep' of the sort which provides private
refuge for the self. Thus, this 'existing' in all its intractable purity is nonetheless
'not an *in-itself* [*en-soi*], which is already peace; it is precisely the absence of
all self, a *without-self* [*sans-soi*]'. Without 'end', neither does the '*there is*' have
an origin in the sense of a constituting or enabling limit, since a 'beginning' or
'starting point' would put us on the pathway to the emergence of a subject as
one who, precisely, takes such a beginning upon themselves (pp. 48–9).

If insomnia is, seemingly paradoxically, 'constituted by the consciousness
that it will never finish', this only points to the fact that the relationship between
consciousness and the anonymous vigilance of the '*there is*' challenges thought
from beginning to end in Levinas's text. If vigilance looks at first glance like a
simple property – or at any rate an irreducible condition – of consciousness,
Levinas nonetheless approaches the question of their precise interaction with
great rigour:

> It can also seem paradoxical to characterize the *there is* by vigilance, as if the
> pure event of existing were endowed with a consciousness. But it is necessary to
> ask if vigilance defines consciousness, or if consciousness is not indeed rather
> the possibility of tearing itself away from vigilance, if the proper meaning of
> vigilance does not consist in being a vigilance backed against a possibility of
> sleep, if the feat of the ego is not the power to leave the situation of impersonal
> vigilance. In fact, consciousness already participates in vigilance. But what
> characterizes it particularly is its always retaining the possibility of withdrawing
> "behind" to sleep. Consciousness is the power of sleep. This leak within the
> plenum is the very paradox of consciousness. (p. 51)

Vigilance does not, therefore, simply give consciousness its essential characteristic. Rather, for Levinas, consciousness arises out of the possibility of its
own remission, asserting itself over the unremitting presence of the '*there
is*' through its capacity for unconsciousness or sleep. As Levinas puts it,
consciousness 'refers to a situation where an existent is put in touch with
its existing' by dint of 'a rupture of the anonymous vigilance of the *there is*'
which comes about through sleep (p. 51). Consciousness may well take part in
vigilance (it is not merely opposed to what vigilance means), but nevertheless

it arises in its specific form through precisely the ability to retreat from vigilance itself. 'Consciousness appears to stand out against the *there is* by its ability to forget and interrupt it, by its ability to sleep', Levinas writes (p. 64). Consciousness is thus a specific 'mode of being', but it also implies a 'hesitation in being' precisely at the moment being is 'taken up' by consciousness. In this sense, if the unconscious operates in tension with consciousness, as it does for psychoanalysis, here the tension is a productive one (unconsciousness as sleep 'is not a new life which is enacted beneath life; it is a participation in life by non-participation, by the elementary act of resting' (p. 66)); although recourse to the unconscious nevertheless marks something like a basic schism in consciousness, since by means of sleep it awakens to being only by dint of a certain turning away from pure existing. While Levinas's argument here participates intriguingly in the entire philosophical 'text' which concerns itself with sleep (one may recall both consciousness's indebtedness to sleep and sleep's status as an outgrowth of consciousness in a long tradition that runs from Aristotle through Enlightenment philosophy right up to the twentieth century and beyond), his claim – one that finds its echo in a certain Blanchot – still seems extraordinary to us. For it suggests that sleep – nothing other than sleep – defines the very conditions of possibility of consciousness. Without sleep there would be no consciousness, no awakening to the 'day'. Consciousness finds its starting-point – it locates itself, as Levinas will go on to suggest – through nothing less than sleep.

In advance of Levinas's major philosophical works, the itinerary of *Time and the Other* moves us from 'anonymous existence to the emergence of subjectivity, to subjectivity's practice, theory and mortality, to its shattering relationship with the alterity of the other person', as the translator's Introduction puts it (p. 2). This establishes at least one aspect of its close relationship to another text by Levinas written around the same time, *Existence and Existents*.[17] Here, Levinas seeks to contest the grounds of the ontological difference in Heidegger, or in other words the distinction between Being and beings, which Levinas chooses to recast with the terms 'existence' and 'existents'. Part of Levinas's project at this time was to leave the 'climate' of Heideggerian thought while not seeking a return to the world of pre-Heideggerian philosophy. In *Existence and Existents* we therefore find Levinas challenging Heidegger's account of thrownness in the world and the ecstatic character of Dasein, in favour of a description of the 'condition' or 'base' from which the subject is posited as an 'event' rather than a 'substantive', as Robert Bernasconi has put it.[18] Bernasconi writes:

> Whereas Heidegger had insisted that Being is always the Being of a being, Levinas sought access to a Being independent of beings. He did this by approaching the relation of beings to Being not as something given, but as an accomplishment. This loosened the tie between Being and beings. Levinas wanted to show that there is existence without existents. (p. xi)

For Bernasconi, whereas Heidegger 'assumed that the human being always already has an understanding of Being and is concerned about Being', thus making the point of departure of Heideggerian thought 'the ecstatic relation, the way the human being lives outside itself as a being in the world', Levinas instead regards the human being in terms of the accomplishment of a 'contract' they make with existence. This entails a specific incision in the '*there is*', a rupture in pure existing, as itself a reaction against the implacable, impersonal vigilance which only comes to be known (however unknowably) through insomnia, and which threatens the very disappearance of the 'world' (pp. xi-xii). Bernasconi makes this comparison in order to suggest how Levinas's philosophical endeavour throughout the late 1940s relates to the prevailing 'climate' of Heideggerian thought. For Bernasconi, then, what is at stake here is Levinas's belief that, in contrast to the Heideggerian themes of the ecstatic character of Dasein and thrownness in the world, 'the value of European civilization lay in its search for a way of surpassing being, and that every civilization that accepts being, the tragic despair it entails and the crimes it justifies, deserves to be called barbarous' (p. x). Thus it is that the trajectory of Levinas's writing from the late 1940s may be described by his translator in terms of the passage from the '*there is*', to the positing of the subject, to the question of responsibility and the other.

In *Existence and Existents*, sleep is once more crucial in thinking the difference between the awakening of consciousness to its day-time concerns and the limitless vigilance of the '*there is*'. Again, insomnia is how Levinas describes this difference:

> The impossibility of rending the invading, inevitable, and anonymous rustling of existence manifests itself particularly in certain times when sleep evades our appeal. One watches on when there is nothing to watch and despite the absence

of any reason for remaining watchful. The bare fact of presence is oppressive; one is held by being, held to be. One is detached from any object, any content, yet there is presence. This presence which arises behind nothingness is neither a *being*, nor consciousness functioning in a void, but the universal fact of the *there is*, which encompasses things and consciousness. (p. 61)

Here, intriguingly, Levinas draws a distinction between attention, which is always oriented towards an object – and which therefore remains the property of a subject – and vigilance itself. This is interesting since it implies that Levinas is a key point of reference in thinking of the vigilance beyond attentiveness to which both Blanchot and Derrida point. Blanchot, of course, calls upon the term in his semi-rejoinder to Bergson in 'Sleep, Night' near the close of *The Space of Literature* (first published in the mid-1950s), where he writes: 'Bergson said that sleep is distinterestedness. Perhaps sleep is inattention to the world, but this negation of the world conserves us for the world and affirms the world' (p. 265). By aligning sleep with an inattentivity to exteriority which in fact serves awakening consciousness, Blanchot seems to draw near to Levinas's idea of sleep as that which, by providing the basis for consciousness to posit itself, reacts to the ever-vigilant '*there is*' that threatens the very disappearance of the 'world'. Given the significance Levinas's text therefore acquires in understanding Blanchot and indeed Derrida on these matters, it is worth quoting *Existence and Existents* at some length:

The distinction between attention, which is turned to objects, whether they be internal or external, and vigilance, absorbed in the rustling of the unavoidable being, goes much further. The ego is swept away by the fatality of being. There is no longer any outside or any inside. Vigilance is quite devoid of objects. That does not come down to saying that it is an experience of nothingness, but that it is anonymous as the night itself. Attention presupposes the freedom of the ego which directs it; the vigilance of insomnia which keeps our eye open has no subject. It is the return of presence into the void left by absence – not the return of *some thing*, but of a presence; it is the reawakening of the *there is* in the heart of negation. It is an indefectibility of being, where the work of being never lets up; it is its insomnia. The consciousness of a thinking subject, with its capacity for evanescence, sleep and unconsciousness, is precisely the breakup of the insomnia of anonymous being, the possibility to "suspend" ... have a night to oneself to undo the work looked after and supervised during the day. The *there is*, the play of being, is not played out across oblivion, does

not encase itself in sleep like a dream. Its very occurrence consists in an impossibility, an opposition to possibilities of sleep, relaxation, drowsiness, absence.
This reverting of presence into absence does not occur in distinct instants, like
an ebb and flow. The *there is* lacks rhythm, as the points swarming in darkness
lack perspective. For an instant to be able to break into being, for this insomnia,
which is like the very eternity of being, to come to a stop, a subject would have
to be posited. (pp. 61–2)

Any reading of Blanchot's *L'Arrêt de mort* (also from the late 1940s, of course)
must surely acknowledge this passage as a possible description of its every page.
For, throughout, we are confronted by a terrifying 'fatality of being' which, for all
that, does not permit us some heroic encounter with 'oblivion' or 'nothingness',
yet which neither lets itself be recast simply as some nightmarish dream.
Throughout, we suffer the 'arrythmic pulsations' of insomniacal jerks between
seeming bouts of unconsciousness, which never quite give rise to the sovereign
moment of empathy or epiphany. Throughout, amid the near-dissolution of the
very terrain of objects and selves, indeed of the 'internal' and the 'external', we
experience the terrifying anonymity of the night which seems to prevail over all.
Throughout, we find every subject (including the reader) pushed to the limits
of what may be posited in its name. One might almost describe *L'Arrêt de mort*
in terms of just this 'reawakening of the *there is* in the heart of negation'. Or, put
differently, one might read Blanchot's text precisely in terms of 'an indefectibility
of being, where the work of being never lets up; it is its insomnia'.

Existence and Existents quickly turns to the theme also broached in *Time
and the Other*: that of consciousness's participation in 'vigilance', despite all
its difference from the anonymous eternity of the '*there is*'. Here, Levinas ties
'the impersonal event of the *there is*' to a notion of 'wakefulness' in contrast
to consciousness. Consciousness, however, participates in this wakefulness
in a particular way. It affirms itself as consciousness precisely because 'it
only participates in it' (i.e. consciousness defines itself through reserving
the right to a temporary withdrawal or partial separation from vigilance).
'Consciousness,' observes Levinas in *Existence and Existents*, 'is a part of
wakefulness, which means that it has already torn into it. It contains a shelter
from that being with which, depersonalized, we make contact in insomnia'
(pp. 61–2). In participating in fundamental vigilance, absolute wakefulness
or the '*there is*', consciousness also tears into it, making for itself a 'shelter' in

the very midst of pure existing's unblinking, anonymous watchfulness. Thus Levinas writes:

> Wakefulness is anonymous. It is not that there is *my* vigilance in the night; in insomnia it is the night itself that watches. It watches. In this anonymous nightwatch where I am completely exposed to being, all the thoughts which occupy my insomnia are suspended on *nothing*. They have no support. I am, one might say, the object rather than the subject of an anonymous thought. To be sure, I have at least the experience of being an object, I still become aware of this anonymous vigilance; but I become aware of it in a movement in which the I is already detached from the anonymity, in which the limit of impersonal vigilance is reflected in the ebbing of a consciousness which abandons it. (p. 63)

In contrast to the unsheltered, unsupported character of insomnia, sleep for Levinas represents an elemental identification with place, allowing being as consciousness to localize itself in a basic way. 'Sleep', he writes, 'reestablishes a relationship with place qua base. ... This surrender to a base which also offers refuge constitutes sleep'. Indeed, the 'position' or site of consciousness is not added after the fact, once consciousness has come into being, 'like an act that it decides on'. Identification with a 'base' does not happen because of the intellectual, affective or volitional powers of consciousness in its given or established form. Rather, 'it is out of position, out of an immobility, that consciousness comes to itself'. Position comes first, as that which enables the very 'positing' of consciousness. Here, in another critical engagement with Heidegger, Levinas writes:

> It is not a question of contact with the earth: to take one's stand on the earth is more than the sensation of contact, and more than a knowledge of a base. Here what is an "object" of knowledge does not confront the subject, but supports it, and supports it to the point that it is by leaning on the base that the subject posits itself as a subject. (pp. 67–8)

For Levinas, place, before being considered in terms of 'geometric space', and before being understood in terms of 'the setting of the Heideggerian world', is to be thought of as a base that 'is not posited' by someone or some entity, but which is instead foremost 'a position'. 'It is not situated in a space given beforehand', an 'earth' with which we make contact as part of the existential drama; rather 'it is the irruption in anonymous being of localization itself' (p. 69).

Here, then, in the midst of a certain reading of Heidegger, we are once more exposed to this extraordinary claim by Levinas, namely that sleep is the constitutive force or enabling limit found at the very origin of consciousness. Sleep, as that which absolutely embraces the 'base' or 'place', sets the conditions for consciousness to emerge as a form of positing, that is on the basis of the 'position' in which it locates itself via sleep. In the fullest sense possible, therefore, consciousness arises or awakens from sleep.

It is important to note that Levinas's characterization of sleep as the basis of consciousness qua 'position' profoundly influences Blanchot's 'Sleep, Night'. Here, we recall that Blanchot writes:

> To sleep badly is precisely to be unable to find one's position. The bad sleeper tosses and turns in search of that genuine place which he knows is unique. He knows that only in that spot will the world give up its errant immensity. The sleepwalker is suspect, for he is the man who does not find repose in sleep. Asleep, he is nevertheless without a place ... He lacks fundamental sincerity, or, more precisely, his sincerity lacks a foundation. It lacks that position he seeks, which is also repose, where he would affirm himself in the stable fixity of his absence, which would be his support. Bergson saw behind sleep the totality of conscious life minus the effort of concentration. On the contrary, sleep is intimacy with the center. I am, not dispersed, but entirely gathered together where I am, in this spot which is my position and where the world, because of the firmness of my attachment, localizes itself. Where I sleep, I fix myself and I fix the world ... My person is not simply situated where I sleep; it is this very site, and my sleeping is the fact that now my abode is my being. (p. 266)

Indeed, Blanchot concludes this passage with a note telling us that 'this is strongly expressed by Emmanuel Levinas (*From Existence to Existences.*)'. It is Levinasian thought, then, that shapes Blanchot's response to Bergson. For while Bergson sees sleep giving rise to a dispersal of 'the effort of concentration', so that the 'totality of conscious life' is given much freer rein in dreams, Blanchot follows Levinas in arguing that sleep facilitates the concerted pulling-together rather than the scattering or diffusion of consciousness.

In *Existence and Existents*, this situation of consciousness's positing can be described in terms of 'hypostasis'. The subject affirms itself, in the etymological sense of finding firm foundation, by locating a ground within the '*there is*' from which a being may arise. Hence, says Levinas, we are authorized to use the term hypostasis, 'which, in the history of philosophy, designated the event by which the act expressed by a verb became a being designated by a substantive' (p. 83). The advent of a being, in other words, resides in just this 'event' – an event in a strong sense – whereby its substantive character arises on the strength of a performative accomplishment, or, put differently, on the basis of its positing. This positing is, then, a kind of *doing* – albeit a 'doing' that does not proceed from the form of being that consciousness 'is', but which instead gives rise to the very possibility of that being. Thus:

> An entity – that which is – is a subject of the verb *to be,* and thus exercises a mastery over the fatality of Being, which has become its attribute. Someone exists who assumes Being, which henceforth is *his* Being. (p. 83)

However, for Levinas hypostasis in fact designates only the 'apparition of a substantive', since 'the suspension of the anonymous *there is*' is only seeming; or rather, it is based on a performance, an appearance, taking the form of 'the apparition of a private domain, of a noun' (p. 83). An entity – the one who exists since he 'assumes Being', the one who is hypostasized – is just the 'subject of the verb *to be*'.

And yet, in a last word on sleep in *Existence and Existents*, Levinas concludes, perhaps somewhat enigmatically, that while we must not 'fail to recognize the event in sleep' (that is, the very event which permits the advent of consciousness as a being), nevertheless 'we must notice that into this event its failure is already written. Fragile sleep, soft-winged sleep, is a second state' (p. 84). Sleep, it would appear, is bound to play second fiddle to consciousness. As that which makes possible consciousness itself, sleep nonetheless seems destined to dwindle in importance, overshadowed by an awakening being which itself provides the basis to recast sleep – perhaps inevitably – as a somewhat derivative and indeed privative form of existence. It is as if consciousness must master, rather than succumb to, that which makes it possible. It must include within itself, as a partial characteristic, that which is in fact constitutive of its being. If in Levinas sleep is inscribed with a different complexity than in the intricacies of the Blanchotian 'text' which readily acknowledges his influence, nonetheless the productive interplay between sleep and consciousness which Levinas describes seems, here, to encounter a certain limit, one which nevertheless also conditions its possibility. Thus, in 'God and Philosophy',[19] the problem is formulated according to a further description which only re-complicates sleep's relationship to vigilance itself:

> Insomnia, wakefulness or vigilance, far from being definable as the simple negation of the natural phenomenon of sleep, belongs to the categorical, antecedent to all anthropological attention and stupor. Ever on the verge of awakening, sleep communicates with vigilance; while trying to escape, sleep stays tuned in, in an *obedience to the wakefulness* which threatens it and calls to it, which *demands*. (pp. 155–6)

Dream of Sleep

Cascando

In Beckett's *Cascando*,[1] a 'Voice' begins, abruptly: '– story ... if you could finish it ... you could rest ... sleep ... not before'. Looking to the past, it continues with broken jerks of language: ' ... oh I know ... the ones I've finished ... thousands and one ... all I ever did ... in my life ... with my life ... saying to myself ... finish this one ... it's the right one ... then rest ... sleep ... no more stories ... no more words ... and finished it ... and not the right one'. Presumably because the finished story is not the right one, the voice goes on, arrhythmically pulsing: 'couldn't rest ... straight away another ... to begin ... to finish ... saying to myself ... finish this one ... then rest ... this time ... it's the right one ... this time ... you have it ... and finished it ... and not the right one ... couldn't rest ... straight away another'. This other inspires a strained confidence: 'but this one ... it's different ... I'll finish it ... I've got it ...'. The 'Voice' does not, however, begin, but instead comes hard on the heels of an 'Opener', whose opening words it breaks in on, perhaps, trespassing on them, perhaps. The 'Opener' opens thus, as dry as dust we are told: 'It is the month of May ... for me'. There is a pause, before the Opener utters a single further word: 'Correct'. Another pause. The Opener then announces: 'I open' (p. 297).

The 'Voice', a trespasser thrown into the open, reborn to the Spring, starts up and hurries on with a dream of sleep and rest. The dream of a sleep that would put all stories to an end. A story to end all stories, this dream of sleep: 'no more stories ... no more words ... come on' (p. 298). Over. Over and over, this dream, from beginning to end of the play.

Meanwhile, the Opener closes, then starts again, opens again. Just as 'Woburn', a third persona perhaps, itinerant sleeper outdoors, falls and rises again, falls to earth and into the waters ('Woburn … same old coat … he goes on … stops … not a soul … not yet … night too bright … say what you like … he goes on … hugging the bank … same old stick … he goes down … falls … on purpose or not … can't see … he's down … that's what counts … face in the mud … arms spread … that's the idea … already … there already … no not yet … he gets up … knees first … hands flat … in the mud … head sunk … then up … on his feet … huge bulk … come on … he goes on … he goes down. … come on' (p. 298)). Over and over. Living on, perhaps. The Opener, meanwhile, balks at those who may say of him, 'That is not his life, he does not live on that', answering to himself, 'They don't see me, they don't see what my life is, they don't see what I live on' (p. 300). And going unanswered, going on, unanswered.

'The state of suspension in which it's over – *and* over again, and you'll never have done with that suspension itself.'

The dream of sleep puts off sleep, casts it out of doors, down and up, down and out, from land out toward the sea, 'night too bright', no cover, no rest, onward to find a 'hole' or 'hollow', 'what's in his head … a hole … a shelter … a hollow … in the dunes … a cave … vague memory … in his head … of a cave' (p. 298). A hole in his head. A hollow. Dream of sleep, impossible dream. Over and over, start again. The Opener opens once more, announces once more 'the month of May. You know, the reawakening' (p. 301). Tired, nearly the end, near-exhausted, the long days of May once more about to close.

Company I: Mind's eye

In Beckett's *Company*,[2] nearly two decades on, another 'three', the very composition of the work, opened thus: 'A voice comes to one in the dark. Imagine' (p. 3). (Whose voice this? And whose voice saying this?). These three make possible whatever may be in the text: 'Use of the second person marks the voice. That of the third that cantankerous other.' (The one on his back in the dark, perhaps.) 'Could he speak to and of whom the voice speaks there would be a first. But he cannot. He shall not. You cannot. You shall not' (p. 4). Here, then, three classes of personal pronoun, let's leave it at that, leave aside counting the personae.

The other scans the dark:

> There is of course the eye. Filling the whole field. The hood slowly down. Or
> up if down to begin. The globe. All pupil. Staring up. Hooded. Bared. Hooded
> again. Bared again. (p. 14)

On the cusp of wakefulness's 'other' (whatever it may be, sleep, insomnia, dreams), sight seems to lose concentration, seems to lose focus, objectless now, overextending itself to fill 'the whole field', losing the distinction between itself and other. Without trajectory, origin or end. As the entire 'globe' becomes nothing but 'pupil', sight stares merely at 'itself', is bared to nothing but itself, which of course it cannot see, cannot accommodate, cannot accomplish, cannot posit or take in. Hooded. Bared. Hooded again. Bared again. The 'eye' that endures the 'dark' thus 'grows more obscure' the longer it 'dwells', until 'the eye closes' and, freed from opening, gives itself over to mental inquiry or introspection. Seemingly. Though, in turn, 'the mind too closes as it were. As the window might close of a dark empty room' (p. 15). Is this the onset of sleep, the beginning of dreams, or the persistence beyond waking thought of an insomnia that won't end? 'Pangs of faint light and stirrings still. Unformulable gropings of the mind. Unstillable' (p. 16).

A vision or a memory would seem to follow, 'say for verisimilitude the Ballyogan Road', where a child in the company of his father is seen 'on the way from A to Z' ('nowhere in particular on the way from A to Z … Somewhere on the Ballyogan Road in lieu of nowhere in particular') (p. 16). But 'out since break of day and night now falling', dark once more descends. Nonetheless, the one on his back in the dark imagines a light, 'at break of day', when a child might 'slip away … and climb' to a 'hiding place on the hillside' (p. 17). 'You lie in the dark and are back in that light', says a voice. The eyes that peer out from a 'nest in the gorge', straining until they 'ache', are forced perhaps to close. 'You close them while you count a hundred.' Memory, onset of sleep, unwinnable struggle against insomnia, which? The eyes 'open and strain again', again and again, counting to a hundred, until 'in the end it is there' – sleep? – light seems to return, 'palest blue against the pale sky', while 'you lie in the dark and are back in that light. Fall asleep in that sunless cloudless light. Sleep till morning light' (pp. 17–18). Once more, sleep, or dream of sleep, sleepless dream of sleep?

The closing eye, seeing as it closes, seeing itself closing; the body arranged 'in supine position or prone' (p. 19), always a matter of *position*, precisely; the wait for sleep, counting the uncountable time, totting up a lifetime's heartbeats in the 'timeless dark', never able of course to reckon, to enumerate in full; uneasy thoughts of daybreak, memories, visions of waking pursuits, plodding on 'from nought anew', lulling one to sleep or to dreams of sleep (p. 27). 'Wearied by such stretch of imagining', 'all ceases', 'he ceases', until, again, 'the need for company' quickens what there is in the dark (p. 31). Given to 'the closed eye in your waking hours', 'by day and by night', the distinction is lost between absorption, dreaming, somnambulance, and rest (p. 30). Each overflows the other. Between sleeplessness and sleep. In the 'dark', mind's activity lessens, becoming ever more slight, perhaps; yet still unstillable, and, as it ever more lessens, perhaps more unstillable still. Though 'supineness become habitual and finally the rule' (p. 46), though the dark never abates even in the midst of shadowless visions, remaining until dawn in this 'position', suspended between sleep and dream of sleep, restless insomnia and fatigued collapse, eyes opening and closing. Indistinguishable dark and light.

Company II: Other voice

Thus, at the centreless centre of *Company*, itself opened by a voice, or rather voice saying 'voice', voice of a voice, at this centreless centre there is 'one on his back in the dark', perhaps. Given in the third person, it seems (each attempt at naming seems to founder). The apparent addressee of a 'voice' that speaks in the second. A voice which says, for example, 'You are on your back in the dark', 'You first saw the light on such and such a day', 'Your mind never active at any time is now less than ever so', and so on (pp. 3–5). The uncertainty of this voice's object of address is soon apparent:

> Though now even less than ever given to wonder he cannot but sometimes wonder if it is indeed to and of him the voice is speaking. May not there be another with him in the dark to and of whom the voice is speaking? Is he not perhaps overhearing a communication not intended for him? (p. 4)

Of whom and to whom the voice speaks, whether to and of the 'one on his back in the dark' or to and of another (in the same dark or in another dark altogether) is a question which must go answered. For while it may seem to apostrophize, to enter into a wholly private exchange (one saturated by

memory and melancholia, even the intimacy of dreams), this voice nevertheless always resorts to the second person in the very structure of its
address. It remains general or impersonal in the formal sense: it speaks to
an unnamed 'You'. This also means, as the text itself wants to insist, that the
voice cannot itself be addressed or spoken *to*, precisely because the question
of whom it addresses, whom it calls to respond, remains irresolvable. And
if the voice indeed speaks *to* another, another still – a possibility which
cannot be discounted – it must therefore also speak *of* another, in a way
which cannot help but alienate and displace the (supposed biographical or
even autobiographical) subject within the narrative space which we might
otherwise think devotes itself to him. Here, paradoxically enough, it is the
apparent immediacy, intimacy or 'inclusivity' of an address in the second
person – 'You' – that forces what may be memory's return or imagination's
upsurge to realise itself in the form of a more or less violent displacement.
Unable to respond to the voice in the second person in which the voice
itself speaks (unable, that is, to reciprocate or communicate), and unable to
register a language or sense of 'self' in the first, precisely because the supposed
biographical content of the voice's remarks – which might otherwise allow for
self-recognition – could very well relate to some other addressee altogether,
the 'one on his back in the dark' is *for just these reasons* condemned to dwell
in the third. 'Could he speak to and of whom the voice speaks there would be
a first. But he cannot. He shall not. You cannot. You shall not': here, the voice
announced by the use of the second person would seem to regain focal control
of the text, although we shall have to return to the question of just who it is
that, a moment beforehand, says 'He'. A prohibition is therefore uttered (but
what is its origin?) which may be meant for the one on his back, but which
may also very well address another still, including quite possibly the reader
him- or herself, who is just as likely referred to by the voice that says 'You'
as any addressee we might find 'in' the text. Thus, one might even say that
the reader as possible addressee is henceforth implicated by and therefore
stealthily drawn into the now uncertain space of the work, as something like
its own innovation (that is, one who is devised on the strength of another's
imaginings). The devising of the reader along these lines – *you*, reader – may
well be constitutive, but, just the same, it once more precludes the possibility
of saying 'I'. Thus, the borders of the text become as dislocated as its 'internal'

space and workings. This sense of dislocation is only reinforced by the one on his back's failed attempt to calculate the 'form and dimensions' (p. 23) of the dark as a *place* that might be demarcated according to a 'unit' of measurement based on the reach or span of a 'crawl' (p. 35). (Indeed, as the text dwells both on its own repetitions and the limits of its memory, setting out each time 'from nought anew' – a phrase which mixes a sense of endless recurrence with that of unprecedented improvisation – it becomes evident that time itself cannot be counted, or counted on, with any more certainty than steps.)

Thus, it is as much due to the 'formal' problem of the voice's uncertain address as because of the vicissitudes of memory, the immersion in dreams, or the encroaching yet unknowable 'darkness' as a metaphor for mental disin-tegration, that the supposed closed space of an autobiographical subject and narrative is incalculably opened, and irreparably dislocated. (If this problem can indeed be separated from those others.) But who, then, says 'You', 'You cannot', 'You shall not'? For that matter, when it is asked whether or 'why' another (another addressee) may reside 'in another dark or in the same' the question immediately imposes itself: 'And whose voice asking this?' Which, in turn, raises another question still: 'Who asks, Whose voice asking this?' (pp. 16–17). To seek to attribute or identify the 'voice' (any voice that speaks in the text) implies that *it* has become the object of address, the object of enunciation *of another*. Which other? To ask the question merely redoubles the problem, since this other that seeks to render an other 'voice' nameable can itself be brought into language – and, thus, to the point of recognition – only as the object of enunciation of *another still*. According to a logic of a certain proliferation – one so fundamentally dislocating that it could never be contained in any one place, including any one text – the very possibility of attributing identity emerges only on condition of a deeply unnameable and ever-retreating (yet never absent) 'deviser' – a 'deviser' of 'company' – that radically replaces the subject or, indeed, the traditional structure of a subject-position. The proposition of a biographical or autobiographical 'self', the possibility of recourse to the first person, the idea of the text's (or the dark's) knowability, and hence its ultimate self-containment or closure, the dream of assigning a name to the voice that speaks – all these aporetic possibilities come into view only via a movement of continual displacement whose origin remains in unfathomable darkness or anonymity. Thus it is that, far from faltering according to some paralysis in the function of the personal pronoun, the text cannot but continue to speak – can hardly stop speaking – from the perspective of this radically originary or constitutive anonymity that collapses or confounds the relations between its three recognizable classes.

Thus the inaugural or inaugurating voice of the text – not that of the 'voice' marked by use of the second person, but instead that of the voice of the 'voice', or in other words that which voices the 'voice' – remains unnameable, unclassifiable. Who exactly 'in' the text says 'he cannot. He shall not' prior to the ominous reintroduction of the 'voice' ('You cannot. You shall not') if the class of pronoun used is not that of the second person? Another voice opens the text, the one which, in uttering *Company*'s very first line, names the voice as 'voice'; and this 'deviser' remains unplaceable within the linguistico-topological field of *Company* to the extent that its utterance flouts the distinctions found among the classes of personal pronoun. In speaking of a 'voice' coming to 'one', the text's inaugurating sentence implies (if read in one way) a certain kind of self-reference, and yet if read differently this might also predicate 'one' as the other or another, blurring the boundary between first and third person while contriving a sense of address that is strongly redolent of the second. (This 'one' is therefore radically and undecidably pluralized in the text's inaugurating moment.) What is uttered in the incipit, then, radically opens the text, and whoever or whatever speaks here remains unplaceable in relation to the voice that it 'names' (as possibly, yet undecidably, its own – a voice, that is, which comes to 'one' perhaps in the sense of coming to oneself-as-oneself). Yet as Badiou, in *On Beckett*, has noted,[3] this unnameable origin of what(ever) may be 'nameable' is a trickier figure than that of the opposite or double or of a formal paradox, since there is always a three-fold configuration – *another still* – which triangulates through opening as much as closing the third side.

The effect more or less repeats itself at the text's point of 'closure'. Here, the final word – 'Alone' – seems on the one hand to imply that whatever company we encounter in Beckett's novella is a mere illusion or delusion, fostered by a disintegrating self confronted with those fragments of memory or dream which, rather than permitting self-recognition, violently displace the 'self' from itself. However, 'Alone' is preceded by a long paragraph given in the second person:

> Thus you now on your back in the dark once sat huddled ... Huddled thus you
> find yourself imagining you are not alone while knowing full well that nothing
> has occurred to make this possible ...From time to time with unexpected grace
> you lie ... So in the dark now huddled and now supine you toil in vain ... Till
> from the occasional relief it was supineness becomes habitual and finally the
> rule ... Till finally you hear how words are coming to an end ... And how better
> in the end labour lost and silence. And you as you always were.
>   Alone.
>
>   (p. 46)

Is 'Alone' uttered by the 'voice' on behalf of another (on behalf of the 'one
on his back'), therefore emerging as the conclusive act of dispossession, the
last instance of alienation, in a text which bars recourse to the first person?
Perhaps. But then again, despite the rhetorical flow in which the text culminates, apparently targeting this last word as its crescendo, what proves that
'Alone' is voiced by the 'voice' which characterizes itself by use of the second?
Of course, it is simply not possible to determine, grammatically, which – if
any – class of personal pronoun provides the context or setting for this stand-
alone word 'Alone'. And therefore it is not possible to know who says it. In
fact, with similar effect to the 'one' referred to in the text's incipit, 'Alone'
(precisely as it stands alone) does not *isolate* but *pluralizes*. In a sense, despite
its 'aloneness' it keeps a sort of company with (and within) itself, albeit of a
kind which – just as the word 'Alone' shares itself undecidably among plural
possibilities – anonymizes. *Company* is thus open-ended at both ends, and
the 'one' and 'alone' (all-one?) that seemingly inaugurate and close the text
reinscribe originary anomymity at the heart of those linguistic possibilities
– and limitations – stemming from the interplay of the different classes of
personal pronoun.

Beckett and Descartes

As John Pilling wrote more than 30 years ago, Beckett 'received no formal
philosophical training' and 'not unnaturally' remained 'sceptical about philosophy's claims to answer the questions it raises'.[4] 'Nothing would be easier
than to dismiss the philosophical dimension of Beckett from our discussions',
writes Pilling, 'except for the crucial fact which is insistently forced upon

us: that he has read, and been attracted by, most of the major philosophers from Pythagoras onwards'. For Pilling, it is Beckett's exposure to Descartes in particular that gives him 'a concrete model from which to seek satisfaction on the fundamental questions, metaphysical, epistemological and linguistic, that philosophy asks'. (As Badiou puts it in *On Beckett*, 'Beckett was raised on Descartes' and 'the reference to the *cogito* is explicit in many texts' (p. 9). However, Badiou sees Beckett as complexly 'reversing' Descartes, while inhabiting his procedure to a significant extent.) Indeed, for Pilling, Descartes's philosophy marks 'the beginning of modern thought' (p. 112) to the extent that it moves away from 'abstract metaphysical system-building' and begins instead 'with one's epistemological relationship with the outside world' (what Foucault will describe as 'the discourse of the exercise'[5] in the first *Meditation*, which vies with the philosophical project of devising a set of propositions forming a *system*). Yet while Beckett accepts Descartes's 'methods' he refuses his 'consolations', insists Pilling (p. 114). Descartes's '*Meditations* seem to echo behind every page [Beckett] writes', but nonetheless the conclusions reached by Descartes's philosophy are rejected. Moreover, for Pilling the supposed 'style' and 'serenity' of Descartes's writing is strongly at issue in precisely those echoes found in Beckett's work, as if the philosophical content and linguistic form of Descartes's texts must go hand in hand, and one cannot be confronted without the other.

It is not too difficult to see in Beckett's figure of the 'one on his back in the dark' a degraded caricature of the Descartes that we encounter in *Meditations*.[6] Beset by the radically doubtable nature of memory, belief, experience and environment, both set about testing the possibility of, as *Company* itself puts it, 'what can be verified', in a spirit of rigorous scepticism which includes at its centre a crucial element of self-doubt. While, of course, Descartes assumes certain apparently irresolvable problems and positions in the interests of advancing a particular philosophical argument, so that the 'serious difficulties' (p. 23) into which he is thrown in the first two meditations in fact allow the grounds to be established for a perhaps more 'serene' philosophy to emerge (a 'serenity' that, as we shall see in the next chapter, Derrida deeply contests), nevertheless the images of Descartes with which we are presented – of a figure unsure whether he is awake or asleep, mistrustful of his senses, uncertain of the dimensions or existence of his body, sceptical of scientific 'truth', and aware that he may continually be deceived by 'some evil mind' (p. 22) – resonate powerfully with the dark and uncertain landscape and linguistic interplay of *Company*. If, as Peter Boxall has argued, it is impossible in *Company* to own one's own life or one's own past, precisely because 'the experience of lived time does not allow for the possibility of gradual accumulation',[7] this fundamental insight resonates with the opening move of the first *Meditation*, not least in drawing out one of its more enduring – if often unacknowledged – problems. For Descartes, it is the entire edifice of one's beliefs accumulated over a lifetime that calls for wholesale investigation, since any false or misguided belief provides a local platform upon which others come to base themselves. Thus, one must go back to the most basic foundations, ruthlessly pruning out not only what is palpably false, but also stripping away all that is in any way doubtworthy. Moreover, this 'general overturning' must, above all, be timely. Thus, while Descartes conceives of his 'project' at a much earlier age, nevertheless he waits:

> to reach such a mature age that no more appropriate age for learning would follow. Thus I waited so long that, from now on, I could be blamed if I wasted in further deliberation whatever time remains for me to begin the project. Therefore today I appropriately cleared my mind of all cares and arranged for myself some time free from interruption. I am alone and, at long last, I will devote myself seriously and freely to this general overturning of my beliefs. (p. 18)

Setting about his task neither too early nor too late, eschewing both undue speed and unwarranted delay, Descartes begins his project *with perfect timing* 'today', in an ideal present unencumbered by youthful haste or melancholic regret. Indeed, if 'the experience of lived time' that is itself responsible for the stealthy accumulation of beliefs is not to interfere with the 'serene' inheritance (and rationally-conducted 'general overturning') of what has been gradually accumulated, this massive undertaking must indeed be realized firmly in the present instant, 'today'. That such a task is paradoxical is of course fairly self-evident, given that some 'lived time' would always have to be taken to correct the 'gradual accumulation' that characterizes the work of time itself. But the problem is compounded here by the fact that the work of the first two meditations, which culminates in Descartes' philosophical breakthrough (*cogito ergo sum*), apparently takes place over two days. Or, at any rate, it occurs as an event during a period of time which seems to straddle the threshold between night and day, mapping an uncertain borderline which drifts and divides precisely where thought vies with dreaming and with sleep. Thus, it is doubly uncertain whether Descartes's thought ever takes place during the day, 'today', in the present tense.

Of course, the story of Descartes' *Meditations* is well known. Writing in an era characterized by the onset of profound scepticism, Descartes chooses not to reassert dogmatically the value or idea of truth, which would be wholly counterproductive in regard to its intention, but instead decides to radicalize doubt, to put it to work with such impeccable rigour that anything which survives the onslaught might open a pathway to certitude. And it is indeed doubt that does all the work here: the very fact that Descartes is *able to doubt* proves to him that there is something or someone there doing the doubting – that someone or something exists and must exist in order to doubt. Doubt, paradoxically enough, turns out to be the very thing that gives rise to certainty. Thus, Descartes is certain that he exists because doubt demonstrates the existence of thought and of a thinking being. Yet, as has often been noted, the affirmation of the cogito is accompanied here by an unwanted effect. The cogito is doubled as subject and object of the *Meditations*, appearing as that which is thought, and as that which thinks. In other words, the cogito is both the end-product of a philosophical investigation based on the radical assumption of doubt, and the prior condition of possibility of this philosophical procedure, without which doubt could not take place. Indeed, at the very beginning of the first *Meditation*, Descartes assumes that he is able to clear 'my mind of all cares' – i.e. to separate and distinguish the *content* of the mind, that which is doubtworthy, duplicitous, 'other', from its essential nature and pure performativity as rational thinking tool – and that it is possible for him to arrange 'for myself some time free from interruption' (even though the meditations effectively proceed as a series of somewhat phantasmic debates and dialogues with unattributed philosophical arguments or 'voices'). Uninterrupted time, a pure present that ultimately emerges as indistinguishable from the pure and uninterrupted presence of a rational self-consciousness – this surely presupposes the principal characteristics of the modern Western subject in its classical guise? In this sense, the very last thing that is doubted in Descartes's *Meditations* is the cogito itself, the one thing that is supposed to withstand the test of doubt in its most robust form. Thus, the cogito is radically dislocated across the uncertain space and time of the first two Meditations, emerging as its own double, both thinker and thought, subject and object of philosophical enunciation. Yet this double is irretrievably fractured and dispersed in the text, since the cogito functions as both unquestioned precondition and resilient end-product of doubt. And there is triangulation once again here, since this effect is not only one of a closed, formal paradox, *but opens the very question of its own origin*: what Badiou might see as the 'third' which triangulates through opening as much as closing (pp. 53–4).

Madness, Sleep

As is well known, in Derrida's 'Cogito and the History of Madness'[1] we find the contested interpretation of Descartes's first *Meditation* taking centre-stage in a lengthy reading which outlines Derrida's reservations concerning Foucault's *Madness and Civilization*. For Derrida, while Foucault seeks to resist forms of discourse that find their origin or context in the precepts and language of reason, by necessity he is also in danger of repeating them. Foucault's project therefore runs the risk of the re-internment or reappropriation of madness – or rather the madness/reason opposition – as an 'object' of knowledge, reasoned inquiry, or clear-headed scholarship. (Indeed, Foucault's determined effort to escape such snares is, as Derrida puts it, at once 'the most audacious and seductive aspect of his venture, producing its admirable tension', but also, 'with all seriousness, the *maddest* aspect of his project' – a sign at once of its failure and success, perhaps (p. 34).) As Derrida argues, 'this attempt to bypass reason is expressed in two ways difficult to reconcile at first glance': namely, a tendency to 'globally' dismiss or universally reject 'the language of reason' in precisely its 'universal rationality', on the one hand; and, on the other, a concerted effort to historicize the emergence and supremacy of its logic and power – *as if it were the very conditions of its historicality that granted it universal or inescapable domination* (including dominance over the conceptual field governing any 'history' of reason or madness, even and perhaps particularly an 'archaeology', as Derrida suggests). Thus, in the opening stages of Derrida's essay we are presented with the constraints that are perhaps inevitably encountered in Foucault's project of a history of madness, and the tensions or contradictions (one might even venture to say, the signs of *madness*) that open up within the field of reason at the very moment Foucault struggles with the task before him.

In question here is not only the manner in which the 'object' of Foucault's interest is produced by way of its empirical determination in a critical discourse which cannot but pretend to transcend the empiricity it wants to analyse. Derrida finds in Foucault's historicism the same effect that in *Of Grammatology* he discerns in the work of Levi-Strauss: namely, a particular event assigned a certain historical significance comes to rely on conditions of possibility that the analysis itself renders universal. Derrida therefore argues that Foucault makes of the violent partition and objectification of madness at once an historical occurrence taking place in the 'classical age' or 'age of reason' inaugurated by developments in seventeenth-century Europe[2]; and yet that the movements and tensions in Foucault's argument also cause 'madness' to appear as effectively a condition of the very possibility of history in general. If history itself is the history of reason (a 'reason' which, Foucault argues, constitutes itself at bottom by a decisive separation from madness), then the seventeenth-century discourse of madness is but an instance in this history, a determinate form that reason takes in a particular setting. The particular circumstances of the 'mad' in the historical period to which Foucault attributes madness itself would henceforth be, in Derrida's terms, only 'a socioeconomic epiphenomenon on the surface of a reason divided against itself since the dawn of its Greek origin' (p. 40). The historical setting of madness singled out by Foucault cannot therefore provide the basis to account for what Derrida calls 'the historicity of reason in general', and thus can be granted neither absolute privilege nor archetypal exemplarity. In particular, if reason was indeed undivided prior to the 'classical age' (an idea Derrida imputes to Foucault), from which time its 'division' – as a profound structural crisis or event – produced 'madness' in its very possibility, then this very same 'classical age' must be, as Derrida points out, only 'secondary and derivative' in relation to reason itself – it 'does not engage the entirety of reason' (p. 42), and therefore cannot provide the basis for narrating the history of reason which in turn supplies the context for the history of madness.

Obviously Derrida does not highlight apparent contradictions in Foucault's project simply to castigate his work as a fall from logic, rigour, sense or reason itself. Instead, of course, he puts in question the very distinction between madness and reason that he sees establishing the grounds of Foucault's argument and structuring its limitations. ('The attempt to write the history of the decision, division, difference runs the risk of construing the division as an event or structure subsequent to the unity of an original presence,' writes Derrida, 'thereby confirming metaphysics in its fundamental operation' (p. 40).) Turning to Descartes – whom he takes as Foucault's exemplary thinker of the classical age which itself becomes responsible for the partition of the mad – Derrida argues that madness is not, for him, the most serious threat to the quest for rational certainty that takes place through a general process of doubting. Indeed, madness is not just a condition of possibility of reason in the sense that it facilitates a certain phase in the process of doubting on its way towards certitude (in fact, as we shall see, Derrida is less convinced than Foucault of the significance of the brief evocation of madness in the first *Meditation*). Madness is, as Derrida shows, more radically a possibility of reason, in the sense that Descartes's argument has to acknowledge the possibility of 'thought' being all the while *mad* as it proclaims the Cogito. For *Cogito, sum* must hold true whether one is mad or sane, enlightened or deceived, insists Derrida. At its most 'proper and inaugural moment' (p. 56) – which is also its most 'hyperbolical' or excessive moment – nothing is therefore less certain than the 'good sense' of the Cogito, since for Descartes's thesis to work, Derrida tells us, sanity is precisely *not* constitutive of its certitude. Rather than seeking to decide in any simple sense between the empirical and the universal as the origin of reason's historicity and madness's partition, then, Derrida shows how, when one turns to the Cartesian heritage, 'thought' can propose or grapple with the determinate, conceptual or historical form of all except the hyperbolic moment that grants its possibility. ('I think, therefore, that (in Descartes) everything can be reduced to a determined historical totality except the hyperbolical project' (p. 57), writes Derrida.) This, perhaps, is the very condition of philosophy itself, its interminable crisis, which is also its historicity in a highly complex sense: 'philosophy is perhaps the reassurance given against the anguish of being mad at the point of the greatest proximity to madness' (p. 59).

All that having being said, by contesting Foucault's reading of the first *Meditation*, Derrida questions the extent to which madness can be separated from other forms of 'non-reason' and thus the extent to which it may be accorded a unique position in the story of reason itself. As 'Cogito and the History of Madness' turns from Foucault to Descartes, therefore, Derrida is quick to note that Descartes generalizes 'the hypothesis of sleep and dream ("Now let us assume that we are asleep")'[3] by means of a kind of hyperbole which, we may surmise, is similar to the hyperbole that for Derrida ultimately grants the possibility of the Cogito's certitude (p. 46). Derrida's essay, as we said a moment ago, culminates in the argument that madness is not the most serious threat to the quest for rational certainty that takes place through a general process of doubting, being instead part of the very possibility of reason and certitude (of the Cogito); but, here, it is also *not* to be taken too hastily as the principal medium for the hyperbolicization that, for Derrida, leads to the crowning moment of Descartes's argument, or at any rate to the deep significance of his thought. Foucault, however, wants to distinguish madness more decisively from other forms of sensory misrecognition such as dreaming. Derrida argues that Foucault treats madness differently from 'dreams and all forms of sensory error', writing as he does in *Madness and Civilization* of a 'fundamental imbalance between madness' and these other forms within the 'economy of doubt' (cited in Derrida, p. 46), and seeking to separate madness from the category of error in general. As Foucault puts it, then, Descartes is unable to 'avoid the peril of madness in the same way he circumvents the eventuality of dream and error' (ibid.). Derrida observes that Foucault wants to read Descartes as suggesting that dreams are limited in their disruptive or disturbing force since they cannot fundamentally constitute, in Derrida's terms, the 'simple and universal elements which enter into their creations' (p. 46). For Derrida, this limitation is, in Foucault's interpretation of Descartes, allied to the limits of sensory error in general. Thus, Foucault writes that, for Descartes, only madness can take 'doubt to the extreme point of its universality'. '"Let us assume we are asleep"' does not cause 'truth' to 'entirely slip out into the night', insists Foucault, while 'for madness, it is otherwise' (cited in Derrida, p. 47). For this reason, argues Derrida, Foucault sees Descartes as sidelining the possibility of delving into madness – or, rather, into the interiority of the experience of madness – since, for the thinking subject to be what it is, madness is an impossibility, whereas dreaming (or other forms of sensory error) palpably is not. Or, as Derrida writes of Foucault's interpretation of Descartes, madness is 'expelled, rejected, denounced in its very impossibility from the very interiority of thought itself' (p. 47). In Foucault's argument about madness, therefore, sleep and dreaming are at once powerfully secondarized as a feature of Descartes's effort to radicalize doubt; yet at the same time – since madness at once takes doubt 'to the extreme point of its universality' but still remains radically impossible for the thinking subject – dreams would seem to represent something of a limit or frontier of doubting as an experience for the Cogito *as such*. If Foucault's reading of Descartes thus ends up in a seeming tangle of contrary possibilities, Derrida seizes on this moment to suggest, quite starkly, that 'Foucault is the first, to my knowledge, to have isolated delirium and madness from sensation and dreams in this first *Meditation*', both in their 'philosophical sense and their methodological function' (p. 47). The implication is quite clear: since this separation which Foucault attributes to Descartes would posit madness as the exclusive medium for the most radical or extreme form of doubt, while at the same time presenting it as a condition that goes entirely beyond the horizon of what may be doubted – since doubt is precisely the constitutive experience or creation of a thinking subject – such a characterization of madness as opposed to dreaming doesn't only lead to philosophical contradictions but, more crucial still, it is sufficiently incoherent to unsettle the boundary which, Foucault argues, maintains the very distinction between madness and dreams in the first place. For if Foucault's reading of Descartes leads to the suggestion that madness is at once doubt's profound limit yet its ultimate scene, this defining tension would weaken the supposed opposition to dreams, since despite seeming to uncover the pathway to deepest doubt, dreams are themselves equally unable to grant access to its very heart, its most intimate 'inside' (according to Foucault's own argument, as we shall see, dreams in Descartes – contra Derrida – should not be taken as the privileged medium of a hyberbolic generalization of doubt). Here, we might note, the state of sleep is, once again, secondarized or diminished in importance, only to return as the repressed, divided 'truth' of the 'other' which had been taken to dominate or supersede it.

Reading Descartes contra Foucault, Derrida is quite explicit about the possibility of separating 'the philosophical sense' and 'methodological function' of madness and dreams in the first *Meditation*:

> Descartes *does not* circumvent the eventuality of sensory error or of dreams, and does not "surmount" them "within the structure of truth;" and all this for the simple reason that he apparently does not ever, nor in any way, surmount them or circumvent them, and does not ever set aside the possibility of total error for *all* knowledge gained from the senses or from imaginary constructions. It must be understood that the hypothesis of dreams is the radicalization or, if you will, the hyperbolical exaggeration of the hypothesis according to which the senses could *sometimes* deceive me. (p. 48)

Here, then, dreams are not to be so easily appropriated or superseded in the way that, for Derrida, Foucault attempts. Derrida continues: 'In dreams, the *totality* of sensory images is illusory. It follows that a certainty invulnerable to dreams would be *a fortiori* invulnerable to *perceptual* illusions of the sensory kind' (p. 48). Dreams are sufficient to allow us to inquire into the characteristic features and, more particularly, the possible limits of sensory error. 'Which are the certainties and truths that escape perception, and therefore also escape sensory error?', asks Derrida. 'They are *simple* and *intelligible* things', such as – by analogy – the colour which painters do not invent, and could not possibly invent, but which they merely use (as something necessarily 'real') to fashion pictorial representations or, in other words, imaginative illusions. Nonetheless, the 'certainty of this simplicity of *intelligible* generalization', as Derrida puts it, in no way proposes or suggests that the senses enjoy any kind of 'invulnerability' to doubt. Instead, as he asserts:

> *All* significations or "ideas" of sensory origin are *excluded* from the realm of truth, *for the same reason as madness* is excluded from it. And there is nothing astonishing about this: madness is only a particular case, and, moreover, not the most serious one, of the sensory illusion which interests Descartes at this point. (p. 50)

Contra Foucault, Derrida goes on to re-read Descartes's subsequent, ostensible insistence on basic realities as a 'juridical' device, one which ventriloquizes the 'astonishment and objections of the nonphilosopher' or 'novice in philosophy' rather than truly representing 'Descartes's final, definitive conclusions' (p. 50). When Descartes thus writes that only an insane person would deny the fact of his own hands or body, he simply pretends to put himself in the position of the astonished greenhorn, as Derrida would have it, precisely in order to move the argument forward, philosophically speaking. And, importantly for Derrida, Descartes appears to dismiss the possibility of madness principally to underline the fact that 'the example of madness is therefore not indicative of the fragility of the sensory idea'. One does not need to be mad to doubt even the most apparently irrefutable evidence of one's senses, and the example of dreaming – 'the experience of sleep and dreams', to borrow Derrida's phrase – succinctly illustrates this:

Descartes then elaborates the hypothesis that will ruin *all* the *sensory* foundations of knowledge and will lay bare only the *intellectual* foundations of
certainty. This hypothesis above all will not run from the possibility of an
insanity – an epistemological one – much more serious than madness.

The reference to dreams is therefore not put off to one side – quite the
contrary – in relation to a madness potentially respected or even excluded by
Descartes. It constitutes, in the methodical order which here is ours, the hyperbolical exasperation of the hypothesis of madness. (p. 51)

On this interpretation, sleep and dreams do not therefore constitute merely a
limited example in contrast to madness which more properly and profoundly
'takes doubt to the extreme point of its universality', as Foucault would have
it. Instead, the 'hypothesis of madness' is itself 'hyperbolically exasperated' by
'reference to dreams'. Or, as Derrida puts it, somewhat more eye-catchingly:
'What must be grasped here is that *from this point of view* the sleeper, or
the dreamer, is madder than the madman' (p. 51). Or, rather, the dreamer is
'further from true perception than the madman' in regard to 'the problem of
knowledge' since, as Descartes's imaginary conversation with the novice is
intended to suggest, madness is more easily dealt with than dreaming when
tackling the question of sensory error in all its profundity. 'It is in the case of
sleep, and not in that of insanity', writes Derrida, 'that the *absolute totality* of
ideas of sensory origin becomes suspect, is stripped of "objective value" as M.
Guéroult puts it' (p. 51). Hence, 'the hypothesis of insanity is therefore not
a good example, a revelatory example, a good instrument of doubt' because
it neither extends across 'the *totality* of the field of sensory perception' nor
functions strongly as a pedagogical tool (and thus a powerful philosophical
instrument) precisely to the extent that it succeeds less well than the example
of dreams in overcoming the resistance of the non-philosopher. For Derrida,
then, Foucault –in his rush to assert an epoch-founding 'factual determination of the concept of madness' (p. 51)[4] – mistakes Descartes's primarily
'juridical usage' of the example of madness in the construction of a particular
philosophical argument. For Derrida, Foucault fails to understand the use of
madness in the first *Meditation* as merely 'a sensory and corporeal fault' that,
while it represents a relatively serious condition for 'all waking but normal
men', is in fact far less serious 'within the epistemological order' than the error
to which we succumb during our dreams (p. 51).

Of course, as those familiar with the basic arguments of Derrida's essay (stated at the outset of this chapter) will appreciate, the madness which Descartes seems to set aside in his 'juridical' usage of its example returns in more radical guise as 'no longer a disorder of the body, of the object, of the body-object outside the boundaries of the *res cogitans*, outside the boundaries of the policed city', as Derrida puts it (p. 53). Derrida describes this 'return' in terms of the movement from 'natural doubt' to 'radical doubt': whereas in the former phase, insanity quickly gives way to dreaming as the principal aid to Descartes's argument, in the latter, it returns more profoundly (on the other side of dreaming, one might say) as a form of madness 'that will spare nothing', that gives no shelter from doubt to ideas either of sensory or intellectual provenance, and that welcomes into the 'essential interiority of thought' that which was 'previously set aside' as mere ailment or physical disorder (p. 52). This is because, as we move through Descartes's *Meditation* from madness to dreaming and back again, *in principle* 'nothing is opposed to the subversion named insanity' (p. 53) where the existence and thought of the Cogito is concerned. Ultimately, nothing can defend against its possibility; indeed, for Derrida this possibility must be admitted in order for Descartes's argument about the Cogito to succeed. Thus, 'Descartes never interns madness ... *He only claims to exclude it during the first phase of the first stage, during the nonhyperbolical moment of natural doubt*', writes Derrida (pp. 55–6). Before the 'historic' separation of a '*determined* reason' and a '*determined* unreason', then, there is *in principle* the 'hyperbolical' or 'mad audacity' of the Cogito which is itself invulnerable to this very same separation. (Seeking to rearticulate Foucault's thesis on his own terms, Derrida goes on to suggest that – on the basis of an extended reading of Descartes's text – the historic internment of the mad might be connected with reason's attempt to articulate and implement itself according to normative discourses, methods and practices which could not tolerate the profound madness at the core of its possibility. And, of course, it is God who in the end protects the Cogito against the madness to which it is otherwise always susceptible, and philosophy which seeks to restrict hyperbole within the 'order of reason' (pp. 58–9), according to a 'philosophical' negotiation which deconstruction must reinvent, says Derrida.) To the extent that Foucault's book misses this point about the 'mad audacity' of the Cogito, however, it itself risks a certain incarceration of madness, and indeed a certain straitjacketing of the Cogito – which Derrida links to a certain 'structuralist totalitarianism' which at this time he wished both to analyse and resist.

In his famous response to Derrida, 'My Body, This Paper, This Fire',[5] Foucault embarks upon a close re-reading of Descartes's text, endeavouring along the way to expose Derrida's argument as too remote from the philosophical ruses and discursive ploys of Descartes's writing. Foucault wants to insist that the way Derrida's argument proceeds is faulty, and that a major flaw to which this leads is the supposition that 'the example of dreaming is for Descartes only a generalization or radicalization of the case of madness' (p. 404). For Foucault, madness and dreaming confront one another in Descartes's text according to an entire scheme of differences which cannot be reduced to the sweep of Derrida's argument (whereby madness is taken to be quickly superseded by the more useful and productive example of dreaming). In particular, focusing on 'the discursive practice' of the first *Meditation*, Foucault argues that Derrida deeply misunderstands Descartes's brief evocation of madness, not treating it properly as part of a 'discourse of the exercise' (p. 410) which intervenes such that the 'test of madness' and the 'test of dreaming' (p. 412), far from functioning as near-identical operations, remain quite distinct in their purpose. Foucault writes that the *Meditations* 'require this double reading' whereby we are confronted with 'a set of propositions forming a *system*, which each reader must follow through if he wishes to feel their truth, and a set of modifications forming an *exercise*, which each reader must effect, by which each reader must be affected, if he in turn wants to be the subject enunciating this truth on his own behalf' (p. 406). The reference to madness in the first *Meditation* is, Foucault argues, part of a distinct process linked to the 'discourse of the exercise' which therefore relates more to the second than the first aspect of this 'reading': 'the meditating subject had to exclude madness by qualifying himself as not mad' (p. 412). 'Once this qualification of the subject has finally been achieved', says Foucault, 'systematic discursivity' is once more allowed to 'take the upper hand' (p. 410) – a process which, indeed, also allows a certain exclusion of madness from philosophical discourse. Here, then, Foucault is seeking to question Derrida's argument about the precise significance of the move from madness to dreaming – and all that it implies – by arguing that the discursive planes and operations of Descartes's text are more complex and differentiated than Derrida allows. Thus, Foucault describes Derrida as 'the most decisive modern representative' of a long-standing 'system' going back to the classical period. This 'system', he argues, is characterized by a tendency to reduce 'discursive practices to textual traces', and to elide 'the events produced therein' in favour of retaining 'only marks for reading'. In Derrida's case, suggests Foucault, the continued dominance of this 'system' may even lead to the invention of 'voices behind texts' (i.e. the philosophical novice whom Derrida conjures up in the midst of the first *Meditation*) in order that the inter-preter may 'avoid having to analyze the modes of implication of the subject in discourses'. The set of tendencies enshrined in this 'system' of interpretation or reading are as much pedagogical as metaphysical, says Foucault. In fact, he links them to the teaching that 'there is nothing outside the text' (p. 416).

As his close reading proceeds, then, Foucault casts doubt on both the development of Derrida's argument (in particular, concerning the move from 'natural doubt' to 'radical doubt'), and the justification for it:

> To hold such an interpretation, Derrida had to deny that it was a question of madness at the point where madness was named (and in specific, carefully differentiated terms); now he has to demonstrate that there is a question of madness at the point where it is not named. (p. 414)

Furthermore, in perhaps the most crucial moment of 'My Body, This Paper, This Fire', Foucault challenges Derrida's idea of the 'mad audacity' of the Cogito, by asserting that 'if the evil genius takes on the powers of *madness*, this is only after the exercise of meditation has excluded this risk of *being mad*' (p. 415) – a risk excluded during precisely the phase in Descartes's text where, according to its discursive function (belonging to the discourse of the *exercise* rather than that of the propositional *system*), 'the meditating subject had to exclude madness by qualifying himself as not mad' (p. 412). By this means, Foucault is therefore able to defend his thesis concerning the exclusion of madness against Derrida's assertion that, in the most 'proper and inaugural moment' of the Cogito, 'nothing is opposed to the subversion named insanity'.

To sum up: in Derrida's interpretation of Descartes, a perceived tendency on Foucault's part to secondarize sleep and dreaming in relation to the supposed exemplarity of madness is significantly reversed. In the process, what Derrida's argument suggests is not only that madness fundamentally and constitutively divides reason (rather than being divided *from* or *by* reason itself). It also implies that Foucault's conception of madness is itself deeply divided, since, in Derrida's reading of his erstwhile teacher, madness at once takes doubt 'to the extreme point of its universality' while yet remaining fundamentally impossible for the thinking subject who is supposedly constituted by just this extreme process or possibility of radical doubt. Moreover, since the distinction which Derrida suggests that Foucault makes between madness and dreaming in Descartes presents madness as at once the unique vehicle for doubt 'at the extreme point of its universality' and yet also a defining symptom of the limits of reason or of the (doubting) Cogito itself, the very 'identity' that madness acquires in Foucault is insufficiently coherent to maintain the distinction between madness and dreams on which Foucault depends. If Derrida is right that Foucault's interpretation of Descartes figures madness as at once doubt's inviolable threshold yet also its most decisive setting, this very same tension upsets the demarcation of dreams, since despite seeming to promise access to radical doubt, dreams do not in fact lead us into its most intimate interiority (Foucault, of course, insists that Derrida's argument concerning dreams as the vehicle for the hyberbolic generalization of doubt should be dismissed). Thus, on the strength of Derrida's readings of Descartes and Foucault, dreams and sleep can no more be divided from madness than madness can be separated from reason. Indeed, since within the very trajectory of Foucault's response to Derrida the exclusion of madness from reason relies in no small part upon its separation from dreaming within the discursive practice of Descartes's text, it would be nothing less than this insufficiently distinguished figure of sleep or dreaming which returns to complicate the ostensibly oppositional character of Derrida's and Foucault's texts.

If in his defence against Derrida's criticisms, Foucault is largely content to pass over sleep and dreaming, granting them merely a supplementary role in Descartes's discursive practice and the Cartesian text's 'modes of implication of the subject in discourses', it may equally be the case that Derrida's own commitment to the significance of dreams might look to some – not least as his career advanced – like the product of an increasing over-indebtedness to the resources of psychoanalysis (despite all that we know about Derrida's repeated attempts to distinguish his project from that of psychoanalytic thought and practice). Indeed, Derrida reconsiders his relationship to Foucault's work, several decades after the publication of 'Cogito and the History of Madness', precisely in terms of Foucault's more dismissive attitude to the psychoanalytic 'text'. "To Do Justice to Freud": The History of Madness in the Age of Psychoanalysis', from the early 1990s, appeared several years after Foucault's death. [6] As Derrida was keenly aware, it therefore allowed him no opportunity to respond. Derrida is, thus, extremely hesitant to reopen their debate in its original form, but instead raises the question of the (resistant) relationship of psychoanalytic discourse to the Foucaultian 'text' on madness. For Derrida, Foucault is unduly hasty in seeking to 'objectify' psychoanalysis historically, failing to see that his own work emerges from an intellectual milieu which cannot so easily extricate itself from psychoanalytic influences. Psychoanalysis, in other words, cannot be reduced to a simple 'object' of Foucaultian discourse, since it must be taken to inform that discourse to some extent; nor can psychoanalysis be partitioned historically by such a discourse if it enters into its own historical conditions of possibility. Foucault's complex and, for Derrida, often contradictory approach to psychoanalysis is re-read in terms of the resistances which psychoanalysis itself offers to a reductive presumption of its self-identity. Indeed, for Derrida, psychoanalysis's resistance of its supposed 'self-sameness' opens the possibility of a certain deconstruction of Foucault. For this somewhat maddening resistance not only challenges the objectification of psychoanalysis as an identifiable historical form but, by extension, provokes once again the question of the very possibility of an 'age' of madness. In other words, the self-difference of the 'psychoanalytic' which, Derrida argues, begins to seep into Foucault's text at precisely those moments he attempts to identify psychoanalysis *as such* threatens to disturb not only his image of psychoanalysis as an 'object' of critical representation, but also the epistemic categories or historical classifications which underpin the Foucaultian project itself. However, Derrida salutes Foucault for acknowledging difficulties in his conception of the *episteme*. For Derrida, such difficulties do not merely give rise to a paralysing impasse in Foucault's work, but instead provide the always heterogeneous and divided resources which make possible the event of thought.

One can only imagine Foucault's response to this essay – it seems unlikely that it would have paved the way for further reconciliation – and one can only guess at the highly exacting text he might have prepared in reply.

Ultimately, I do not wish to adjudicate the dispute between these two writers. But I mention the third of these three texts forming a sort of Foucault-Derrida dossier, only to point out that their disagreement or divergence largely centred on incompatible notions of what difference or division might mean, in theory and practice. Whether or not Derrida is insightful about the treatment of Descartes (or, for that matter, psychoanalysis) in Foucault's writing – and it would be peremptory to deny the validity of Foucault's response to 'Cogito and the History of Madness' out of hand – nonetheless Derrida's affirmation in '"To Do Justice to Freud"' of the always plural, non-unitary, or divisible resources which make possible thought as *event* not only militate against Foucault's overhasty dismissal of deconstruction as merely a pedagogy devoted to the mantra that there is 'nothing outside the text' (clearly, for deconstruction, these resources cannot be reduced to merely a textual economy). Perhaps more significantly, the emphasis which Derrida places on the constitutive importance of self-difference, put to work in the powerful resistances at play in every text, every event, every 'history', reminds us of the very dispute we have just 'read', where what is in question is not only the image of madness/reason as non-self-identically split and doubled – an image arising from a deconstructive argument that Foucault strongly contests – but also, and more particularly, the heterogeneous force of a madness that, in its very exclusion or separation, cannot distinguish itself entirely from that which (according to Foucault) it supposedly is not. Such resistances, including this (maddening) resistance to the conceptual determination of madness, may doubtless be attributed in a variety of different ways: here, we might add sleep and dreaming to the series of names for that constitutive difference at work in every 'origin'.

Fall of Sleep

An 'equal world'

In *The Fall of Sleep*,[1] Nancy describes an 'equal world' of sleep. 'Everything reverts to the general equivalence in which one sleeper is worth as much as any sleeper … All sleepers fall into the same, identical and uniform sleep' (p. 17), he writes. From this point of view, sleep is not merely the great leveller, sweeping away all the distinctions and discriminations of the day, smoothing out disparate 'passions, sorrows, and joys' in an undifferentiated atmosphere of 'darkness' and 'silence'. As that which is 'shared since unshareable' (p. 45), sleep would also seem to entail the possibility of a radical openness to the other beyond the normative ethics of a welcoming subject or received models of socio-political exchange. For Nancy, such openness may perhaps be figured in terms of the happy intimacy of lovers, whereby sleep as a sinking-down-deeper into the 'loving spasm' suspends what is most intimate 'at the limits of the dissolution and disappearance of their very harmony' (p. 18). (The unshareable sharing which occurs in the midst of sleep may also be glimpsed, Nancy suggests, in the long-forgotten, communal sleep of 'our ancestors'.) Nonetheless, such intimacy-beyond-intimacy is a complicated affair, since lovers' bodies 'insidiously disentangle, however intertwined they can sometimes remain until the end of sleep' (p. 18). Upon awakening, the 'joy' that has been 'eclipsed' by a period of sleep may suddenly return, yet waking sexual communion is not just a matter of restoring the simple closeness that becomes, at the very least, complicated during sleep.

In this section of his book, suddenly and without warning, Nancy inserts a portion of text taken from Derrida's *Glas*,[2] which in turn includes a passage clipped from Genet's *Miracle of the Rose*. Here, Derrida writes of the 'separation' or 'comma' between 'excitement, and I' that is reinstated upon waking alongside one's lover. Awakening desire punctuates the relation of the 'self' to itself: the alliterative refrain of the 'I' and its 'excitement' implies the equality of these two expressions on either side of the pivotal mark which separates them. This confrontation of the newly stirring 'I' with its desire amounts to ('is equal to', says Derrida) a sort of 'decollation', a detachment or ungluing; but also, in this strange economy of equivalences, it provokes 'a sublimating idealization that relieves what is detached'. In an exalted state of 'indecision', the awakened subject quivers with desire, the desiring 'self' oscillates, vibrates, percusses with itself on the threshold of its own tremulous excitement. As the kiss which gives expression to this 'ideality' takes wing, however, we are presented with a curious scene: glued to his lover during sex, Genet nonetheless imagines the possibility of 'a slight twinge, that decollation of a subtle glue' which might accompany his lovers' awareness of a world beyond their embrace (and which, in effect, permeates Genet's own imagination, despite – or perhaps because of – the coming rapture).

Nancy responds to this rather brusquely inserted passage by returning to the theme of the 'forgetting' brought on by sleep, which itself entails another intimacy whereby 'there is nothing to take or keep, nothing to win or save: everything, on the contrary, to let go' (p. 19). It is as if the letting-go that happens during sleep – the insidious disentanglement of slumbering bodies, however entwined they may remain – is placed in contrast to 'that decollation of a subtle glue' that always remains possible during waking intimacy, indeed which perhaps *produces* the very possibility of such intimacy, precisely in the form of an 'excitement' that asserts its equivalence to the 'I' (or for that matter, constitutes its appeal to the other) only by dint of the irreducible potentiality of separation, friction, trembling vibrancy. (Indeed, the more-or-less violent ungluing and re-sticking into Nancy's text of the citation from Derrida/Genet – a cut within a cut, one might say – turns this passage of *Glas/Miracle of the Rose* into an example of what it seems to speak about.) Sleep is, then, a particular kind of letting-go, the suspended momentum of bodies unencumbered by friction, which differs from – although it is hardly the polar opposite of – a certain 'decollation' of desire. Sleep is the relaxation of tension, not as mere 'ease', but rather through 'a very subtle conversion … into the intensity of relaxation that physics calls inertia' (p. 19). Sleep prolongs and transforms the pleasure given us during the abrasions of passion, precisely by means of the dissolution that such passion bears within itself. 'Sleeping together comes down to sharing an inertia', writes Nancy:

> an equal force that maintains the two bodies together, drifting like two narrow boats moving off to the same open sea, toward the same horizon always concealed afresh in mists whose indistinctness does not let dawn be distinguished from dusk, or sunset from sunrise. (p. 19)

For Nancy, then, sleep puts into suspension the unequal or frictional play of forces and fortunes which gives us the possibility of theft as much as of sex (as he himself puts it, sleep leaves us 'nothing to take or keep'). Paradoxically, its profound unshareability provides an image of strange and unworldly commonality beyond, for instance, all forms of secular assembly or religious congregation. Radically uninterested in a division of spoils, sleep renders all equal. Its inertia leaves hanging all differences. Waking intimacy, in contrast, gives us not only the scenography of sexual passions, but also the possibility of daylight robbery.

In these terms, we need to think hard about what may be the two most striking features of Nancy's book: first, as we shall see, its relationship to a series of frequently unacknowledged philosophical sources; second, and relatedly, its seeming refusal to evaluate the specificity or distinctiveness of the various forms of thought it inherits. Is Nancy guilty of intellectual theft, while at the same time putting to the sword precisely the exchange-value of the booty? Does the critical practice of *The Fall of Sleep* amount to a case of daylight robbery? Or is its seemingly wilful disregard for property more the work of a thief in the night? *The Fall of Sleep* – treating as it does a 'topic' at the very limits of philosophizing – was received at the time of its publication as 'Nancy's most lyrical, most beautiful work', 'as much a nocturne as a treatise', 'exemplary of Nancy's practice of finite thinking – thinking without concepts, categories and other philosophical machinery'.[3] These plaudits provide a ready means to explain the book's technique or manner of working, bringing together its deep resistance to all the scholarly operations of philosophy 'proper' and its stylistic attunement to its subject-matter as powerfully interrelated gestures. But such praise for Nancy's 'sleep book', itself bordering on the lyrical, surely demands that we ask of this text just where the limits of philosophical engagement may lie?

Falling asleep: Philosophical drifts

Nancy's ruminations on sleep frequently evoke precisely those texts in the philosophical tradition upon which we have concentrated. At times, his writing appears to endorse as much as put in question some of the principal notions about sleep which one might link to a heritage which includes, say, Aristotle and Kant. For instance, we find echoes of Kant's (and, indeed, Hegel's) dismissive remarks on sleepwalking[4] in Nancy's rather sweeping critique of the world today as a world 'without sleeping or waking', a world deeply somnolent and somnambulant at once, a world increasingly at variance with the rhythms of nature, one that has become a seemingly endless expanse of urban-industrial landscape, an horizon-less complex of interminably floodlit and essentially insomniacal-anaesthetized '24/7' living, where migrating birds 'are thrown off course by the intense halo of light that big cities project into the sky', and where workers are 'knocked out' in a mere parody or caricature of sleep (pp. 38–9). Here, interestingly enough, just the sort of discrimination or differentiation that Nancy himself associates with waking life is foregone, so that – perhaps paradoxically – the analysis on offer would seem to draw on all the resources of the night to make its point about the seemingly unbreakable domination of the day (without, for all that, working up a critical dynamics of this situation in the way that, say, Blanchot makes possible). For, as Nancy himself says, it is sleep itself which 'knows only equality, the measure common to all, which allows no differences or disparities' (p. 17), putting into suspension nothing less than 'the time of differentiations' (p. 21). (Here, we find a striking opposition between day-time as the enabler of every distinction and night as the source of all-engulfing undifferentiation, one that for Nancy leads all the way back to Hegel.[5])

The memory of Kant (among others) is also recalled where Nancy reprises the idea that sleep 'functions to suspend all functioning' (p. 6). For here, we are reminded of Kant's understanding of sleep as 'a wise arrangement of nature for exciting the power of life through affects related to involuntary and invented events, while bodily movements based on choice, namely muscular movements, are in the meantime suspended'. Sleep, in other words, offers the living being rest and recuperation – indeed, it re-stimulates life – without the attendant risk of bodily self-harm that is potentialized by the suspension of a wakeful and alert consciousness. Nevertheless, Nancy's contention that sleep dispossesses us of all functional ability except 'the function of sleeping, which perhaps is not a function' puts sleep itself into an aporetic situation vis-à-vis thought. For here sleep becomes, if not a function to end all functions, a function which nonetheless works to interrupt precisely the functionality of which it must necessarily be a variety.

There are veiled reminders of other thinkers, too. For instance, Nancy elsewhere writes that, during dreams, thought comes to 'play freely, indistinctly distinct, in the expanse of nowhere' (p. 25). This is less of a Freudian echo than one might think (dream-thoughts are not, for psychoanalysis, simply the product of free-play). As one reads on, Nancy comes to associate sleep with 'inattention' and 'noninterest' of a kind which, for him, perhaps even calls forth death (pp. 41–2). Thus, the expansive non-selectivity of the sleeper's imagination recalls Bergson's idea that, whereas in waking life all 'accumulated experience' found in the memory is rapidly 'compressed' so that it can centre on and explain a particular stimulus, during sleep this 'narrowing' of perception and interpretation is much less marked. Instead, for Bergson, the 'tension' that characterizes the waking mind makes way for 'extension'. (Blanchot, remember, observes that for Bergson 'sleep is distinterestedness' or perhaps even 'inattention to the world'.) Indeed, very early on in *The Fall of Sleep*, Nancy strikes a Bergsonian note when he suggests that slumber involves 'the co-presence of all compossibilities' (p. 7). Equally, one can hardly help thinking of Bergson when Nancy writes: 'In sleep, the mind abandons itself to the body and disperses its location through it, dissolves its concentration into that soft, almost disjointed expanse' (p. 35). For Bergson, of course, the part played by the external stimuli which still impact upon the bodily senses during sleep is critical to the understanding of dreams as precisely an expression of the interplay between sensation and memory rather than of a deep-seated unconscious at work. Such stimuli, for Bergson, 'rise and spread' amid a 'wild phantasmagoric dance', one that is controlled far less by the imposition of day-time logic or reason. Of course, Bergson does not think of dreams as simply the product of an unrestricted 'game' taking place. They are constituted, instead, by the degree to which past memory and present sensation are able to combine. Nevertheless, in Bergson's account of sleep, the visions forged in the sleeper's imagination are much more a matter of a certain dispersal of

conscious concentration and consequently a greater – or at any rate different –
subjection to the bodily senses, than they are a product of the mind's descent
into its own unconscious depths. Bergson, of course, argues that the dream is
in fact 'elaborated almost in the same way as perception of the real world' – that
is, through the combination of memory and sensation. However, as we have
seen, this interplay works differently while asleep. Dreams equal nothing less
than the 'entire mental life minus the effort of concentration', an effort which
limits or narrows interpretation in a necessarily swift and thus semi-automatic
way during wakefulness. For this reason, Bergson suggests that the dreaming
mind is in fact hyper-alert while the waking mind is, in comparison, just a
little somnolent. In other words, rather than constituting merely a privative
version of full consciousness, such a mind is intrinsically more awake than
wakefulness itself. When Nancy speaks of 'the always possible imminence of
night in broad daylight' (p. 23), or of dreaming as 'like waking, similar to it' (p.
25), or of a 'soul' that in 'waking … ceaselessly dozes' and 'in sleeping … wakes
and watches' (p. 36), we therefore detect myriad echoes of Bergson, as well
as of Blanchot (echoes of Aristotle and of Hegel, too, since in the preceding
sentence Nancy writes that the 'soul animates sleep as well as waking' (p. 36)).

Indeed, *The Fall of Sleep* teems with gestures towards the Blanchotian
text. Nancy's recounting of the story of Morpheus and Alcyone powerfully
recalls the *arrêt de mort* of J. in the first part of *Death Sentence*. As she
dreams of her vanished husband, writes Nancy, 'Alcyone moves her arms
as she sleeps and wants to embrace Ceyx, but it's air she embraces' (p. 8),
just as, in *L'Arrêt de mort*, J.'s body, mistaken for a corpse, expels a horrible
gasp: 'a sort of breath came out of her compressed mouth' and 'almost at the
same time – I'm sure of this – her arms moved, tried to rise'.[6] In *The Fall
of Sleep*, Morpheus's bidding is none other than a suspension of life/death.
As the lovers – one living, one dead – are transformed into kingfishers by
his kiss, Morpheus's gift to Alcyone and Ceyx is 'metamorphosis of life into
death and again into life, into life stolen, into life flown away and suspended
on the waves' (p. 9). This is doubtless a happier version of *l'arrêt de mort*
than Blanchot's. A few pages later, Nancy speaks of sleep as that which
goes beyond phenomenology,[7] showing itself 'only in its disappearance, its
burrowing and concealment' (p. 13). The reference to 'burrowing' surely
recalls that passage in *The Space of Literature* where Blanchot speaks of

Kafka's *The Burrow*. Here, he writes that 'to construct the burrow is to open night to the other night'. For Blanchot, in a way that is markedly different to Nancy's thought, to seek the 'bad' intimacy of pure self-enclosure in the total repose of sleep is in fact to expose oneself to the dreams which, beyond the limits of self-control, inevitably expose one to the 'outside' (since otherwise total separation would lead to the fatal demise of the very same 'self' in question, a self seeking to defend itself absolutely). To 'burrow' in or 'burrow' down is therefore to expose the self to the limits of itself, the outside *of* itself in the 'other night'. For Nancy, however (for whom a certain kind of self-enclosure makes possible rapture itself), such 'burrowing' or 'concealment' brings, somewhat enigmatically, 'a disposition of intentions and aims as well as the fulfilment of sense' (p. 13). 'Sense, here, neither fulfils nor enlightens', Nancy nonetheless tells us; instead, beyond the threshold of the phenomenological, it 'overflows and obscures signification, it makes sense only of sensing oneself no longer appearing' (p. 13). It is possible to pull a little harder on the thread Nancy leaves here. On the occasions where he talks about sleep and vision or sight in *The Fall of Sleep*, one senses Nancy's indebtedness to 'Dreaming, Writing', Blanchot's essay on Michel Leiris. Reflecting on the dreams of Leiris, as we've seen, Blanchot ties together the abyssal scene which sees the dreamer's gaze move toward the impossible spectacle of its 'self' and an incessant vigilance-beyond-vigilance found in the very 'deep' of sleep. This abyssal turning back of the dream upon itself occurs *as if* the aporetic spectacle of a gaze's movement toward the vision of its 'self' were being repeated, endlessly, otherwise. It is as if the hyper-vigilance – the vigilance beyond all possible vigilance – that this astonishing scene conjures in fact recurs as the most fundamental limit of dreaming. For Nancy, the 'divinity' of sleep entails a profound openness to 'this *ex nihilo* that light first drove back to the heart of darkness in the movement by which it sprang from it' (p. 24). Sleep, in other words, opens onto the nothing that existed before the bursting forth of light in creation worked to partition its undifferentiated expanse, re-describing it as mere darkness, figurelessness, absence of form or thing-hood. Nancy thus writes:

> What the sleeper sees is this eclipsed thing. He sees the eclipse itself: not the fiery ring around it, but the perfectly dark heart of the eclipse of being. But

> this darkness is not an invisibility: on the contrary, it offers the full visibility of what, in front of me – that *in front* where every image comes to be imagined, every color to shimmer, every outline traced – there is no more "in front" and everything is made equivalent to "in back" or to "nowhere". There is no share of the visible, consequently there is no invisible either. (pp. 24–5)

The impossible-interminable spectacle of the 'self' at (or, rather, *as*) the very limit of dreams is here transfigured, as the sleeper's eye is swept into a cosmic abyss which in fact defines both the limit and the more original possibility of vision, appearance, being itself. Interestingly, Nancy chooses to conclude *The Fall of Sleep* by citing a Baudelaire poem, 'Le Gouffre' ('The Chasm') (pp. 47–8):

> On the backdrop of my nights God's knowing finger
> Draws an unceasing nightmare with many faces.
> I am afraid of sleep as one fears a huge hole
> Full of vague horror, leading no one knows where;
> I see only infinity from every window,
> And my spirit, ever haunted with vertigo,
> A numb feeling yearning for nothingness.

In the fall of sleep, one sees nothing but 'the absence of all vision and visibility' (p. 48) – that is, one sees the engulfing *impossibility* of a 'share of the visible'. We do not go into the night, into sleep, 'with our eyes closed', says Nancy. Instead, we see 'that we see nothing and that there is nothing to see, seeing sight clinging to itself', which 'is like seeing the invisible, surely, but is only like its other side or its negative. To sojourn in just that other side, not to try to discern the invisible, that is the blind task of sleep.' To 'see' without discerning the invisible, beyond visibility's 'share', constitutes sleep's 'blind' vigilance.

There are obvious shades of Blanchot in other parts of Nancy's book. His contention that the 'I' of the dream is not the 'I' that sleeps is echoed in Nancy's observation that 'this *I* that sleeps can no more say it sleeps than it could say it is dead ... it is another who sleeps in my place' (p. 5). However, Nancy's idea that the fall of sleep is characterized by an utter loss of distinction between inside and outside, belonging and non-belonging, myself and other, relates complexly to Blanchot's writings. During slumber, Nancy tells us, 'I myself become indistinct ... I coincide with the world ... "I" exist only in that effacement of my own distinction' (p. 7). This reprises the idea of an irreducible alterity – a sort of inseparable anonymity, if you like – entering in as a crucial element in the experience of sleep. Yet, perhaps, it does not so powerfully evoke that structuring difference, beyond or before both the subject and signification, which for Blanchot gives us the *dynamics* of sleep in its complex relationship to waking life. Nancy's text thinks differently about the 'outside' and the interiority of sleep than, say, Freud's account of the persistence of anxiety during dreaming; although, in psychoanalysis, it is precisely such anxiety that arises as the powerful remainder of a sustained connection to the world unregulated by the conscious 'I'. For Nancy, enduring anxiety is not really the upshot of the fall of sleep, a 'fall' which is, notwithstanding, a 'fall inside myself', a 'fall to where I am no longer separated from the world by a demarcation that still belongs to me all through my waking state … I pass that line of distinction, I slip entire into the innermost and outermost part of myself, erasing the distinction between these two putative states' (p. 5).

Here, then, it is the question of what sleep does to the 'outside' of itself – or vice versa – that is crucial in understanding the operations of Nancy's text in relation to those he inherits. For instance, Nancy's critique of the seemingly inexorable rise and persistence of day-time, which he thinks occurs at the expense of the natural rhythms of sleep, depends on a set of thematic or conceptual contrasts which perhaps acquire less critical force than Blanchot's evocation of an 'interminable day', simply because they are capable of a less intense critical interplay. In Blanchot, would-be perpetual day in fact gives way somewhat unwittingly to an 'other night' beyond a simple night-time of rest serving the 'day' in the ordinary sense, an 'interminable day'/'other night' which signals, decisively, 'the threat of the outside where the world lacks'. Thus, the intellectual architecture of Blanchot's writing on sleep seems more critically developed in terms of the complex understanding it offers of precisely this 'other night' of an 'interminable day'. The sophistication of Blanchot's text derives, ultimately, from more complicated interactions between 'day' and 'night', inside and outside, self and other, than are found in much of Nancy's writing; interactions which leave a powerful remainder (here, something like a 'lack') still at work 'outside' the apparently engulfing play of indeterminacy that Nancy associates with sleep.

As we have already suggested, Nancy's thinking of sleep continues to engage with the 'Ur-text' of Aristotle. For Aristotle, you will recall, sleep is characterized as the rest or relaxation that a being possessed of 'sense-perception' gives to itself, in particular to aid digestion and well-being. This is in contrast to other types of sense-deprivation which happen in a less intrinsic manner, for instance through a surprise or chance occurrence (such as that which might cause us to faint), or due to some impact on a more trivial organ of sense (for example, pressure applied to blood vessels in the neck). Sleep, on the contrary, has its 'seat in the primary organ with which one perceives objects in general', as Aristotle puts it. Thus, at bottom, 'sense-perception' – far from resigning its power whilst abandoning itself to sleep – conserves and extends itself, precisely via its own remission or seeming withdrawal. One therefore thinks of Aristotle[8] when reading Nancy's contention that the fall of sleep 'is not a loss of consciousness but the conscious plunge of consciousness into unconsciousness, which it allows to rise up in itself as it sinks down into it' (p. 8). In a more obvious reference to Aristotle, just a few pages later, Nancy contends that 'fainting is done without the consent of the "I," which, by contrast, usually assents to sleep and desires it' (p. 12); while in the earliest passages of his book, the mention of 'lethargy', 'fatigue', 'drowsiness', 'relaxation' and so on as sleep-inducing sensations undoubtedly gestures towards an Aristotelian lexicon. However, for Nancy, 'the truth of this immersion' of consciousness into the unconscious is not, as in Aristotle, that which allows us to account for sleep *philosophically speaking*: that is, as both the 'object' and expression of philosophical reasoning. Instead, it is that which 'overflows and carries away any sort of analysis' (p. 8) (including, presumably, psychoanalysis as much as Aristotelian philosophy), precisely because this same 'immersion' is part of the process whereby the self itself loses all distinction, including those distinctions that would permit its analytic powers or the constitution of analysis itself. Falling inside myself in sleep, 'I' lose all separation and differentiation in regard to the 'world', indeed I lose control of the very demarcations that constitute 'me' throughout my waking life. However, through this process of elision that causes all distinctions to fall away, my 'self' is not just restored to a simple, primordial unity of the kind that might be dominated by an idealizing metaphysics of the subject. The interruption or suspension of all those demarcations which in fact constitute the 'self' far from leads to the possibility of full self-realization or self-sufficiency on the part of a sovereign 'I' as classically construed. For the dizzying fall into the 'equality' of sleep is so profound that it leaves no delimited terrain to master, no self-identical ground over which to preside, no bounded unity to partition or acknowledge, no 'place' to occupy. 'No longer being one's own, no longer properly being in relation to the self-ness of oneself', writes Nancy, the sleeper is therefore 'more deeply and more obscurely' immersed 'in self', 'in such a way that the question of "one's own" tends to disappear (Am I really me? Am I actually what I am, what I have to be?)' (p. 12).) Thus the 'self' experiences neither a process of self-constitution nor one of self-representation, which when put together would see it fated to the philosophical problem of its own partitioning as an 'object' of (self-) knowledge. Instead, it is exposed to the all-engulfing event of self-replacement in the very return to 'oneself' during sleep, a 'return' that marks not so much the moment of self-fulfilment as a giddying fall back into what looks like a persistent and inconcludable state, a state which nevertheless cannot be set aside from the very grounds – or, rather, the very question – of 'one's own' possibility. Here, though, the self-beyond-self that awaits us in sleep is not to be thought of merely as a submerged origin, a forgotten wellspring, a lost foundation. Rather, the self-beyond-self that arises in sleep is nothing less than the unworldly expression of a night which always remains ahead of us, or which at any rate drifts so disorientingly across our lives, overwhelming every distinction awoken by 'the day', that we can never simply put it behind us. '"I" do not make a self, for "I" do not return ... I fall asleep and at the same time I vanish as "I"', writes Nancy. This disappearance, he adds, amounts to a loss of distinction which also engulfs the possibility of '"you" singular or any entanglement in an "us" or a "you" plural' (p. 11). Thus, sleep overruns every distinction between 'you' and 'I', indeed between 'you' singular and 'you' plural, between the other and all others. Once more, we are in the midst of a 'sharing' beyond any allotted 'share', an overpowering abandonment or fall in which the constitutive work of difference or alterity seems to realize itself in rapturous implosion. The critical potential of the coming night's constitutive possibility is thus recast in terms of this engulfing dissolution.

There are further shades of Aristotle in Nancy's idea that 'sleep is itself a force that precedes itself and that carries its power forward into its action. If I'm falling asleep, it's because already sleep has begun to take control of me and invade me before I sleep, before I've begun to fall' (p. 3). Here, sleep would seem to induce itself more or less deliberately, through something of an internal movement within 'me', or rather within the complex space of that which constitutes 'me' as such. Sleep is not taken by surprise (unlike that which causes us to faint), but instead prepares for itself, for its own coming, before itself and by itself. However, in this very same movement, sleep is tasked with outmanoeuvring and overcoming the conscious 'me' who nevertheless courts it through controlled and sometimes elaborate gestures of invitation and submission. This complexity, whereby sleep induces itself before the inducements which induce it (without which, it would be mere fainting), casts a shadow over the idea of sleep as the simple instrument of a sovereign being possessed of 'sense-perception'. It is as if Nancy locates, in the very distinction which allows Aristotle to particularize sleep in relation to other forms of sense-deprivation, a certain monstrosity, a hybridity, indistinction, or non-differentiation which makes of sleep a sort of empty agent of its own necessity. Drawing the 'subject' into an exasperating circle, sleep emerges as a counter-force to the force which in fact forces it or gives it force (i.e. 'sense-perception'). It becomes an effect which nevertheless mediates its own mediation, or which at once produces and obliterates its own grounds. Slumber, from this perspective, emerges less as a simple substrate or prop for dreams (as themselves in some way the expression of living sense). Instead, sleep becomes, as Nancy puts it, the product of 'that which exists underneath and itself exists on nothing else' (p. 23). For him, this makes sleep a matter of the 'night' since, in contrast to wakefulness or the 'day', it is that which does not separate, divide, differentiate or distinguish, consequently failing to establish the grounds even for itself, even as it grounds itself on nothing but itself. This realm of night, then, ushers in an underpinning subterraneanism that underpins nothing, not even itself, but which nevertheless exists as a world of undifferentiated '*substance*' beyond '*accident* or *attribute*', as Nancy puts it – a realm 'which is entirely its own, belonging to no other subject or support, to no authority of validation or justification' (pp. 23–4). Thus it is that, far from simply aiding digestion in the Aristotelian sense, sleep for Nancy sees the sleeper feeding upon himself. 'Like animals that practice hibernation,' Nancy writes, 'the sleeper feeds on his reserves. He digests himself, in a way' (p. 6). The slumber of sense-perception is at once a matter of self-preservation but also, in Nancy's reformulation of Aristotelian thought, a dizzying plunge into a certain groundlessness (to boot, one that can't be dismissed as mere accident or privation), according to which the 'self' is restocked only at its own expense, reconstituted only through the prospect of an immeasurable fall or, rather, a wholly vertiginous transformation ('everything is reabsorbed into me without allowing me to distinguish me from anything' (p. 7)). Robbing Peter to pay Paul, the 'economic' rationale Aristotle attributes to sleeping is subjected to a maddening twist. 'We put ourselves to sleep … No-one puts himself to sleep: sleep comes from elsewhere' (p. 29): Nancy's meditation on sleep recasts this seeming paradox in terms of the aporetic conditions of the sleeping self. Yet what remains in question is whether any more can be said of the interplay between this self-beyond-self and the 'elsewhere' that pervades sleep – an 'elsewhere' that is, no doubt, unavoidably enigmatic, but which perhaps becomes less powerfully so as alterity is swept into the abyss of self-abandonment that characterizes sleep.

The other of sleep

In sleep, Nancy writes, I 'belong only to myself, having fallen into myself, and mingled with that night where everything becomes indistinct to me but more than anything myself' (p. 7). At once, everything is reabsorbed into 'me' during sleep, in a way that dissolves all boundaries between myself, the 'other' or the 'world'; yet, at the same time as this apparently limitless expansion seems to occur, 'myself' is utterly recast as other of itself: a 'oneself' beyond itself. For Nancy, the experience-beyond-experience of sleep – as total repose in a fathomless indeterminacy – makes possible a certain 'sheltering' from all the discriminating and divisive conditions of the day, including those that give rise to 'knowledge, techniques, and arts of all kinds', 'all manifestation … all phenomenality' (p. 14). Thus, in the midst of his discussion of the Kantian thing-in-itself that the sleeping 'self' seems to have become, Nancy cites Hegel's *Philosophy of Mind*: 'Sleep is the state where the soul is plunged into its undifferentiated unity – waking, on the other hand, is the state in which the soul has entered into opposition to this simple unity.'[9] Setting aside whether Nancy's treatment of Hegel via this brief allusion is at all satisfactory, for sure Nancy wants to rethink such a 'unity' beyond itself, or beyond the more conventional understanding of its meaning: a 'unity' is traditionally dominated by the force that allots it as such, giving it every semblance of integrity, while at the same time contradicting the claim to self-sufficiency upon which it must be based. Thus, Nancy remarks that the sleeping self-beyond-self draws close 'to its most genuine autonomous existence', an existence which 'should rightly be called absolute: *ab-solutum*, it is detachment from everything', releasing itself 'even from any relation to its own detachment' (p. 14). Since just this 'relation to its own detachment' normatively secures a 'unity' as nevertheless always constituted by dint of a more or less forceful process of differentiation, for Nancy the *ab-solute* sleeping self attains a more profound autonomy in the 'pure' event of a total eclipse or implosion which detaches it from even its own detachment. The 'presence' of the sleeper is therefore that of 'the thing in itself' which is simultaneously 'a thing of no-thing' (p. 15). This absolute abandonment of the self to itself (which is also total abandonment of itself) opens the possibility of a 'strange peace', writes Nancy, one which he wishes to affiliate to a certain experience of rapture rather than mere 'stupefaction'.

But is it possible to speak of the pure otherness of this rapturous abandonment? Throughout *The Fall of Sleep*, as we have seen, Nancy suggests that 'shared since unshareable' sleep gives rise not just to an 'equal world', but to a profound exposure to the 'other'. For him, this exposure is less apparent in the waking experience of intimacy, which amid all its desires seems unable to dispense with the possibility of 'decollation' (detachment/ungluing), a decollation that in fact impedes self-abandonment at the very same time that it makes the 'I' more or less equivalent to its own 'excitement' (to return to Nancy's citation of Derrida/Genet). Instead, such exposure may be glimpsed in the inertia of sleeping lovers whose disentangling bodies, freed from all friction, share suspended momentum. It is as if, at its most radical point, alterity relinquishes its own force, suspends itself utterly or perhaps opens itself at last to the 'other' of itself. If, as Nancy puts it, 'day is always "another day"' or 'in general, the other of the same' (p. 21), sleep is for him the other of this 'other', an other beyond all differentiation as such.

Would such an 'other' embrace or resist its *own* status as 'other of the same', which Derrida tells us every absolute other must be? Another, related question: would this 'other' free itself from even those structuring differences that are deeply recalcitrant or unresponsive to the work of differentiation? Put differently, would this be an 'other' beyond the irrecuperable play of *différance* as, precisely, differentiation's own excess or 'other'? In 'Violence and Metaphysics',[10] Derrida suggests that the 'other' as absolute, that is as a term without necessary relation, would be the (absolute, absolutely self-same) same, and therefore not what it is: namely, other. In this text, Derrida also conjures the spectre of Parmenides, for whom the infinitely other must still be other *than*, and thus 'no longer absolved of a relation to an ego' (p. 126). Such a relation would nevertheless confound its infinite or absolute otherness and, indeed, divide its identity precisely as given in the absolute form. Indeed, to the extent that the infinitely other would have to be 'absolutely not the same', it would have to be ultimately non-self-same, 'other than itself', and thus not 'what it is', therefore 'not infinitely other', etc. As Derrida puts it, crucially: 'the other cannot be absolutely exterior to the same without ceasing to be other' (p. 126). (He goes on to assert the obvious corollary that 'the same is not a totality closed in upon itself', but rather constitutes a possibility fundamentally marked by, and yet unable to 'enclose', alterity.) This brief précis alone prompts us to ask more questions of Nancy's book. For it is not so much that the question of the 'other' is simply pushed to its limits amid Nancy's various evocations of the problem of sleep. It is also that this question is put somewhat at risk, just where the 'other' is not fully put in question. Losing as it does so much critical force except as an expression of the self's abandonment to itself, the question of the other precisely *drifts*. It would seem that, in the fall of sleep, there is no constitutive (or, for that matter, de-constituting) process beyond or outside of the self's rapturous dissolution; by extension, one wonders whether there is any possible criticality, any heteronomous mode or movement of thought, which could take hold outside of the all-engulfing terms which accompany this abandonment of the 'self' to itself. Indeed, one senses that such effects of self-abandonment may not limit themselves simply to the experience of sleep that Nancy wants to describe as necessarily beyond description. They might also illuminate the specific dimensions of Nancy's own engagement with a certain philosophical inheritance, one that *The Fall of Sleep* may well wish to liquefy. Without first subjecting this tradition to the rigours of a deconstructive thinking and reading poised between philosophical acknowledgement and critically transformative possibility, however, Nancy's vision of total eclipse hazards just the kind of inertia that 'keeps a body in momentum so long as no friction or surrounding matter comes to oppose the pursuit of its trajectory' (p. 19).

Notes

Introduction

1 Ray Meddis, *The Sleep Instinct* (London: Routledge and Kegan Paul, 1977), p. i. Further references will be given in the body of the text.

2 Meddis does acknowledge that sleep also assists survival in the sense that it preserves energy and heat, but he is quick to reassert that, over and above these subsidiary benefits, inactivity is the principal means by which sleep preserves existence. The function of sleep in connection with heat retention and thermoregulation is discussed variously by J. Allan Hobson and Jim Horne, and in Stickgold and Walker (eds). (See notes below.)

3 Meddis spends much of the rest of this frequently very funny book sitting up with elderly ladies who knit or read through the night, tuning in to late-night radio phone-ins to hear inveterate insomniacs bemoan their condition, spending long hours assessing the sleep-deprived as they try to maintain concentration while undertaking mind-numbingly boring tasks, and reporting on the hallucinations of marathon non-sleepers, one of whom flees the room after seeing an enormous gorilla bearing down on him. Without at all putting in question his mental state, one begins to wonder about Meddis's social life during this period.

4 In fairness to Meddis, by the end of the book he begins to mellow, saying that he would not endorse the widespread use of the scientific techniques whose development he not only foresees but advocates and encourages! (He doesn't discount, though, using them on those individuals for whom sleep is some sort of 'problem'.)

5 See Plato, *Laws VII*, in *Complete Works*, ed. John M. Cooper (Indianapolis: Hackett Publishing, 1977). All references in this section are to 807e–808e, pp. 1475–6.

6 For an interesting account of just such a 'disciplinary' politics of sleep, see Simon J. Williams, *The Politics of Sleep: Governing (Un)consciousness in the Late Modern Age* (Basingstoke: Palgrave Macmillan, 2011). This includes sections on what Williams calls 'fast' capitalism, and on the 'biomedicalization' of sleep. On the history of sleep, another interesting title is A. Roger Ekirch's *At Day's Close: Night in Times Past* (New York and London: Norton, 2005), which via a

wealth of historical evidence argues that humans in broadly the pre-industrial, pre-capitalist era used to sleep in two distinct spells during night-time: a first sleep which began a couple of hours after dusk, followed by a waking period of one to two hours, and then a second sleep. Throughout this waking period people were relatively active and indeed interactive. Ekirch suggests that references to the first and second sleep started to disappear throughout Western society during the late seventeenth century, beginning with the urban upper classes in northern Europe. This was partly due to improvements in domestic and street lighting, which lessened the need or desire to retire early, but it was also due to a historic shift towards time-conscious or time-efficient ideologies of all sorts.

7 In the work of J. Allan Hobson, for instance, the concept of psychosis remains important as a way to describe what happens during dreaming, whereby the brain basically withdraws certain chemicals – one is tempted to say, drugs – which are known to block or reduce psychosis in waking life. While this analysis is undoubtedly scientifically based, one wonders what happens when a term such as psychosis is retained in a thesis which deeply questions psychological and psychoanalytic paradigms of interpretation and conceptual frameworks.

8 Alongside the work of J. Allan Hobson, see also for instance Jim Horne, *Sleepfaring: A Journey through the Science of Sleep* (Oxford: Oxford University Press, 2006), especially pp. 9–10. Here, he writes: 'Surprisingly, relaxation is not just an absence of behaviour, but an advanced activity requiring a particularly intricate brain.'

9 Meddis thus also describes the superficial sleep of water-based mammals. See also Jim Horne, *Sleepfaring*, pp. 1–7, which describes the way dolphins sleep 'one-side' of the brain at a time.

10 J. Allan Hobson, *Dreaming: An Introduction to the Science of Sleep* (Oxford: Oxford University Press, 2002), p. 2. All further references will be given in the body of the text.

11 As we shall see, this approach perhaps finds echoes in Bergson's understanding of dreaming around a century earlier, although Hobson is frequently insistent that the neurophysiology of sleep and dreaming has little to do with the influence of sensory stimulation from the outside world, and instead results from changes in brain activity that are largely in-built and spontaneous.

12 D. Kuiken, 'Theories of Dream Function', in *The Neuroscience of Sleep*, ed. Robert Stickgold and Matthew P. Walker (Burlington: Academic Press, 2009), p. 295.

13 See the editors' Preface to the above volume, p. xiii. Here, they also write that slow progress in sleep research in part reflects the fact that 'there does not seem to be a single mechanistic pathway to the generation or termination of sleep'.

14 The citations included in this section of my introduction reprise fully referenced quotations found in each of the chapters of this book.

15 William Watkin, *The Literary Agamben: Adventures in Logopoiesis* (London and New York: Continuum, 2010). Further references will be given in the body of the text.

16 Of course the grounds for such a project lead back to Heidegger, though they are far from exhausted by his work.

17 Plato, *Symposium*, trans. Michael Joyce, in Plato, *The Collected Dialogues*, ed. Edith Hamilton and Huntingdon Cairns (Princeton: Princeton University Press, 1961), 205b, p. 557.

18 For Agamben, if *poiesis* is 'a means in sight of an end' while *praxis* is in contrast 'an end without a means', it is gesture which 'breaks the false alternative between ends and means', presenting 'means which, as such, are removed from the sphere of meditation without thereby becoming ends' (Giorgio Agamben, *Infancy and History: On the Destruction of Experience*, trans. Liz Heron (London: Verso, 1993), pp. 154–5). As William Watkin notes, in his discussion of this aspect of Agamben's work, this 'definition of a means without determinate ends' in fact forms 'the basis of Agamben's presentation of form-of-life as a new mode of thinking', notably in his later book *Means Without End*. See Watkin, *The Literary Agamben*, p. 58.

19 While *poiesis* cannot of course simply dispense with *techne*, nonetheless 'there is no guarantee that *techne* will result in poiesis or the flashing bloom of truth', as Watkin puts it (p. 75).

20 Giorgio Agamben, *The Man Without Content*, trans. Georgia Albert (Stanford: Stanford University Press, 1999), p. 69.

21 Here I allude to Agamben's own declaration, as follows: 'Poiesis, poetry, does not designate here an art among others, but is the very name of man's *doing*, of that productive action of which artistic *doing* is only a privileged example' (*The Man Without Content*, p. 59).

22 As Watkin puts it, after long discussion: 'Poiesis is rhythmical structure. It dictates how human being exists in the essentiality of chronological time and space as continuum', although it, too, 'determines how, at various points, being breaks with the continual and enters into the ecstatic ...' (p. 192). Part of the reason for its rhythmicality/arrhythmicality might indeed follow from the fact that, as Watkin argues, 'the very structure of poiesis [exists] as an alternate and complementary mode of thinking to that of the metaphysical tradition' (p. 197).

Chapter 1

1 Throughout this section I refer to Aristotle, 'On Sleep', trans. J. I. Beare, *The Complete Works of Aristotle, The Revised Oxford Translation*, Vol. I, edited by Jonathan Barnes (Princeton, NJ: Princeton University Press, 1984), pp. 721–8. Page references will be given in the body of the chapter. The translation of 'sense-perception' here gives rise to questions of the kind I go on to suggest.

2 See note 7, below.

3 In his subsequent treatise 'On Dreams', Aristotle begins with a highly involved argument leading to the conclusion that 'dreaming is an activity of the faculty of sense-perception, but belongs to this faculty *qua* imaginative' (p. 730). Moreover, the explanation for dreaming arises in part from the fact that 'even when the external object of perception has departed, the impressions it has made persist, and are objects of perception' (p. 732), especially as such impressions sustain themselves by prolonging their influence upon the emotions. Dreams are more or less coherent or weird in relation to normative 'sense-perception', says Aristotle, based on the extent to which the 'heat generated from the food' causes excessive 'movement' during sleep, which, as it disturbs the blood, disturbs also the images or impressions of which dreams are made. (Too excessive a disturbance, however, obliterates the possibility of dreaming since the images cannot form to any degree of coherence.) The dream-image is thus 'the remnant of a sensory impression taken when the sense was actualizing itself; and when this, the true impression, has departed, its remnant is still there, and it is correct to say of it, that though not actually Coriscus, it is like Coriscus' (p. 734). However, the dream itself is neither, strictly speaking, exactly the same as the image in general (since images may be formed outside of the dream, even during sleep, where they may impress themselves upon the perceptual faculty in a more direct way from the external world – for instance, lamplight, or a dog's bark); nor is the dream's content, properly speaking, thought, not even 'true thoughts' which may nonetheless arise during sleep. Instead, the 'dream proper is an image based on the movement of sense impressions, when it occurs during sleep, insofar as it is asleep' (p. 735).

4 A somewhat different account of the 'biological' or 'physiological' basis of sleep occurs in Plato (although these terms obviously remain rather anachronistic). Here, the eyes – 'the first of the organs to be fashioned by the gods' – are treated as the conduit of a certain 'fire' which is 'not for burning' but which is instead intended to cast a 'gentle light' that connects the 'visual stream' of the eye to the 'light' of the external world, through a process in which 'like makes contact with like'. During the night, however, 'the kindred fire' departs, and thus the visual

stream is 'cut off', unable to connect to that which is 'like' itself. 'No longer able to bond with the surrounding air, which now has lost its fire, it undergoes changes and dies out', not only bringing sight to an end, but inducing sleep itself: 'For when the eyelids – which the gods devised to keep eyesight safe – are closed, they shut in the power of the internal fire, which then disperses and evens out the internal motions', so that 'a state of quietness ensues' which presages sleep. However, to the extent that 'some strong motions remain, they produce images similar in kind': that is to say, dreams. See 'Timaeus', 45b–46a, Plato, *Complete Works*, ed. John M. Cooper (Indianapolis: Hackett Publishing, 1997), pp. 1248–9.

5 Jacques Derrida, *The Animal That Therefore I Am*, ed. Marie-Louise Mallet, trans. David Wills (New York: Fordham University Press, 2008). Further references will be given in the body of the chapter.

6 It would no doubt be possible to write an entire treatise on the significance of the term 'awakening' throughout the 'text' of philosophy. For instance, in a short text on the subject, Samuel Weber has indicated the importance of awakening in Walter Benjamin's writings. (See Samuel Weber, *Benjamin's –abilities* (Cambridge, MA., and London: Harvard University Press, 2008), 'Awakening', pp. 164–75). As Weber puts it:

> "Awakening" – *Erwachen* – is his final attempt to meet the challenge he had outlined in the early programmatic essay ['On the Program of the Coming Philosophy' (1916)]: articulating the "non-synthesis" between concepts that would bring together "thesis and antithesis" in a relation that would not be subsumptive or reductive of their constitutive differences. (p. 167)

For Weber, what Benjamin refers to as the 'supremely dialectical breaking-points of life' are thus to be conceived of as distinct from the power of the negative that underpins the Hegelian dialectic, and must be construed instead in terms of a spatio-temporal determination – a '*place*' – which cannot be, as Weber puts it, 'negated and absorbed by the movement of the concept' (p. 167). 'Such breaks', he writes, are, however, 'for Benjamin not primarily negative or privative in character.' Instead, they 'constitute privileged moments of what, in the following note, he [Benjamin] describes as a "constellation of awakening"' (p. 167). Here, Weber argues, Benjamin distinguishes his notion of awakening from that of the Surrealists, who remain too in thrall of the dream and thus neglectful of 'history'; and yet Weber also notes that Benjamin is quick to criticize Jung for a tendency to overly separate awakening *from* the dream. In these terms, Weber suggests that Benjamin wishes to understand awakening precisely in its relationship to the dream, whereby separation itself defines this very same relation. Weber writes:

It is this *relating through separation* or as separation that characterizes what he calls the "constellation." This could indicate how a certain "non-synthesis" could nevertheless relate concepts to one another while preserving their differences and without subordinating them to a totalizing continuity or unity. (p. 168)

Furthermore, it is from just such a non-sythesizing 'constellation' that 'knowability' – rather than knowledge *as such* – may be derived. As Weber points out, knowability here names not so much the abstraction of a generalized principle as 'a temporal possibility that always exists *now*' (p. 168), albeit a 'now' that remains located in a 'place' – ultimately irreducible to the self-presence or transcendence of a subject – which is itself defined by the impossibility of full actualization, absolute self-determination or self-grounding.

Knowability as a form of potentiality cannot be reduced to a prefatory stage in the transition towards the acquisition of knowledge in a full or proper sense. Instead, its 'distinctive structure', as Weber puts it, is to be understood precisely in terms of an awakening that may be distinguished from the normative conceptual duality of 'consciousness' and 'unconsciousness', emerging instead as a highly singular experience or movement which remains transformative without being goal- or end-oriented:

Awakening must therefore be investigated on its own terms, as a distinctive experience, and not simply as a transition from the dream to being-awake, from unconsciousness to self-consciousness. (p. 169)

In Benjamin's writing on Proust, therefore, Weber detects the suggestion that awakening is not merely one experience among others, but that it perhaps defines the structure of experience itself. Moreover, Benjamin indicates that such awakening exists as the condition of every 'historical presentation' – that is, both as its origin and as the very possibility of a transformative movement *away* from this origin. 'In its restorative, repetitive, never-fulfilled movement the "origin" is, Benjamin concludes, a thoroughly "historical" phenomenon', as Weber puts it (p. 170). In this reading, history is thus made possible by the recursive advent of the singular or, in Derrida's terms, by an always originary iterability which utterly transforms as it repeats: awakening. This movement of history construed in terms of the 'distinctive structure' of awakening is iterable, then, less in terms of legible recursions of the past than by dint of an always potentially irrecuperable or irreparable exposure to the future. Moreover, in Proust, the 'distinctive temporality' of awakening is, for Weber, profoundly linked to a certain locatedness, embodiment, or spatiality: one always awakens *somewhere* (spacing is always temporal, and vice versa; or, as Weber puts it, 'space as extension strives to move away from itself and in this striving it becomes time, which in turn becomes the measure of movement' (p. 173)). This 'somewhere', however, is never simply a self-contained or self-identical place; rather, it is always caught up in the 'distinctive structure' of awakening which in fact establishes its possibility. In Weber's terms, 'the singularity of spatio-temporal positioning' (p. 172) always opens onto an alterity according to whose movement its 'setting' is at once articulated and 'disarticulated' in turn. And this inescapable situation (i.e. that of the spatio-temporal) deeply disturbs the harmonious certainties both of waking-up and falling-asleep. Awakening in Proust is thus, in Weber's terms, something like a 'movement of dislocation ... of stretching to fit the room' which 'not merely accompanies awakening but constitutes it' – awakening to a 'room' that does not 'merely contain' but which instead emerges as the 'stage for a play that is a fragment rather than a complete work: a stage where something comes to pass, a passage-way, perhaps, but one that is not going anywhere' (p. 175).

7 In *Creative Evolution*, doing something rather different with the terminology in question, Bergson writes that 'the humblest organism is conscious in proportion to its power to move *freely*. Is consciousness here, in relation to movement, the effect or the cause? In one sense it is the cause, since it has to direct locomotion. But in another sense it is the effect, for it is the motor activity that maintains it, and, once this activity disappears, consciousness dies away or rather falls asleep.' (p. 123). Or, again, by way of another fascinating complexification of terms, Bergson speaks of 'those outer stimuli which act on the sensibility of the animal as irritants and prevent it from going to sleep. The plant is therefore unconscious. Here again, however, we must beware of radical distinctions. "Unconscious" and "conscious" are not two labels which can be mechanically fastened, the one on every vegetable cell, the other on all animals. While consciousness sleeps in the animal which has degenerated into a motionless parasite, it probably awakens in the vegetable that has regained liberty of movement, and awakens in just the degree to which the vegetable has reconquered this liberty. Nevertheless, consciousness and unconsciousness mark the directions in which the two kingdoms have developed, in this sense, that to find the best specimens of consciousness in the animal we must ascend to the highest representatives of the series, whereas, to find probable cases of vegetable consciousness, we must descend as low as possible in the scale of plants down to the zoospores of the algae, for instance, and, more generally, to those unicellular organisms which may be said to hesitate between the vegetable form and animality. From this standpoint, and in this measure, we should define the animal by sensibility

and awakened consciousness, the vegetable by consciousness asleep and by insensibility' (p. 124). Several pages on, Bergson writes: 'We have already said that animals and vegetables must have separated soon from their common stock, the vegetable falling asleep in immobility, the animal, on the contrary, becoming more and more awake and marching on to the conquest of a nervous system' (p. 143). However, just a little earlier, with perhaps less respect for specific distinctions, he says the following: 'Regarded in what constitutes its true essence, namely, as a transition from species to species, life is a continually growing action. But each of the species, through which life passes, aims only at its own convenience. It goes for that which demands the least labour. Absorbed in the form it is about to take, it falls into a partial sleep, in which it ignores almost all the rest of life' (p. 142). Elsewhere, however, Bergson talks of the lower form of life being the species or individual who think of themselves alone (behaving as if the general movement of life does not, first of all, pass through. . . .). Hence, whichever species manages to retain the greatest degree of wakefulness towards other life-forms automatically attains superiority. See Henri Bergson, *Creative Evolution*, trans. Arthur Mitchell (Modern Library, Random House, 1944).

8 Derrida here cites Martin Heidegger, *Being and Time*, trans. John Macquarie and Edward Robinson (New York: Harper and Row, 1962), pp. 62–3.

9 Immanuel Kant, *Anthropology from a pragmatic point of view* in *Anthropology, History and Education (The Cambridge Edition of the Works of Immanuel Kant)*, eds Günter Zöller and Robert B. Londen (Cambridge: Cambridge University Press, 2007), pp. 227–429. All further references will be given in the body of the chapter.

10 Kant is not alone in his (philosophical) disdain for sleep-walking as a malign anomaly. In Hegel's *Philosophy of Mind*, it is asserted that: 'The only way in which the animal organism in sleep is still related to the external world is breathing, this wholly abstract relationship to the undifferentiated element of air. With particularized externality by contrast the healthy human organism in sleep no longer stands in any relation. If, therefore, a man in sleep becomes active outwardly, then he is ill. This occurs in sleep-walkers' (G. W. F. Hegel, *Philosophy of Mind*, trans. W. Wallace and A. V. Miller (Oxford: Oxford University Press, 2007), p. 65).

11 Herschel Farbman, *The Other Night: Dreaming, Writing, and Restlessness in Twentieth-Century Literature* (New York: Fordham University Press, 2008), p. 3. All further references will be given in the body of the chapter.

12 See Sigmund Freud, *The Interpretation of Dreams*, trans. Joyce Crick (Oxford: Oxford University Press, 2008). Freud argues that the dream '*is the guardian of sleep, not its disturber*' (p. 180). (All further references to this text will be given in

the body of the chapter.) Here, dreaming preserves sleep by negotiating potential interruptions from external stimuli in a variety of ways, using the dream either to deny them or to incorporate them in a way that is compatible with continued slumber. Furthermore, sleep guards the dream against its most self-destructive potential in the sense that the paralysis of the motor function during sleep protects the slumberer against the possibility of real harm (to himself or others) posed by the unconscious as it goes 'rampaging upon the scene' (p. 371). Here, Freud does not consider cases of violent acts done by somnambulists.

13 In *The Interpretation of Dreams* the dream of the burning child, which to some might seem simply traumatic at first glance, nonetheless momentarily prolongs the father's sleep against the full recognition or recollection of his offspring's death (he dreams his child is alive once more). See pp. 330–1; 348; 373–4.

14 In *The Intepretation of Dreams* Freud writes, rather smugly, 'I have no longer had a real anxiety-dream myself for decades' (p. 382).

15 Throughout this book, we will continually return to this issue of a withdrawal into 'self' during sleep versus the ongoing connection to the world that occurs in dreams, through a number of readings of texts running across the continental tradition, including those by Freud, Bergson, Blanchot, Levinas and Nancy.

16 Farbman argues that the dream-work which itself makes possible the dream as 'a particular *form* of thinking' in Freud is nevertheless profoundly unaffected by the 'interests' it supports or expresses, i.e. those of the unconscious wishes at work in the dream. Thus, the dream-work is not itself the upshot or initiative of any subjective agency, even at some non-conscious level. The dream-work, in essence, neither thinks nor feels. It simply 'restricts itself to giving things a new form', as Farbman puts it (p. 39): that is to say, it produces transformations on the material which constitutes dream-thoughts, doing so with dispassionate relentlessness, unguided by judgement, calculation, or responsibility. Thus, as Farbman tells us, 'Freud's theory depends upon this indifference to influence in the heart of the dream' (p. 40). At the origin of dreaming – in the very conditions of possibility of dream-thoughts – we therefore find the radical absence of a subject. To put it differently, something deathly is to be imagined as a non-present remainder at the very core of the dream. Or rather, something like death-beyond-death, something beyond the very possibility of the death of a subject, beyond both consciousness and unconsciousness. Something like the dream that for Blanchot goes before or beyond the day-driven sovereignty of 'I sleep'.

17 G. W. F. Hegel, *Philosophy of Mind*, trans. W. Wallace and A. V. Miller (Oxford: Oxford University Press, 2007). Further page references will be given in the body of the chapter.

Chapter 2

1 See Henri Bergson, 'Dreams', in *Mind-Energy*, trans. H. Wildon Carr, intro. Keith
  Ansell Pearson, (eds) Keith Ansell Pearson and Michael Kolkman (London:
  Palgrave Macmillan, 2007), pp. 82–105. All further references will be given in
  the body of the chapter. It is worth noting here that Aristotle himself observes
  that not 'every image which occurs in sleep' is necessarily a dream. Instead, 'some
  persons ... actually perceive sounds, light, savour, and contact: feebly, however,
  and, as it were, remotely. For there have been cases in which persons while asleep,
  but with eyes partly open, saw faintly in their sleep (as they supposed) the light
  of a lamp, and afterwards, on being awakened, recognized it as the actual light
  of the lamp; while, in other cases, persons who faintly heard the crowing of
  cocks or the barking of dogs identified these clearly as they awoke' (Aristotle,
  'On Dreams', trans. J. I. Beare, *The Complete Works of Aristotle*, The Revised
  Oxford Translation, Vol. I, edited by Jonathan Barnes (Princeton, NJ: Princeton
  University Press, 1984), pp. 734–5). Once more, the legacy bequeathed by
  Aristotle to the philosophical tradition is evident here.
2 One semi-resonance with Freudianism in Bergson's essay consists in the fact
  that he suggests the sleeping mind is more active and far-ranging than waking
  thought, which is really only half-alert to its own experience. In *The Interpretation
  of Dreams*, of course, Freud critiques those that see the dream as 'only a fragment
  of our psychical activity' (p. 64), and in this respect he perhaps draws close to
  Bergson, where the latter argues that the dream, although specific in its nature,
  is nonetheless connected to the 'entire mental life'. Of course the differences
  between the two thinkers are ultimately very great, but there is something here
  which perhaps makes them differently 'modern', or at any rate which places both
  Freud and Bergson in striking contrast to a prevailing, late nineteenth-century
  'scientific' understanding of dreaming as merely a partial and defective form of
  consciousness.
3 In this essay, Bergson describes the 'light-dust' and constantly shifting 'colour
  blotches' which play on the eye when the lids are closed, along with 'the slight
  modifications which are ceaselessly taking place in the circulation of blood
  in the retina' and 'the pressure which the closed lid exerts upon the eyeball,
  causing a mechanical excitation of the optic nerve'. In a thinly veiled reference to
  Shakespeare's *Hamlet*, but probably also ironically to Romantic understandings of
  dreaming, he contends that these are 'such stuff as dreams are made of' (p. 83).
4 In 'On Divination in Sleep', Aristotle writes that, during sleep, 'even trifling
  movements seem considerable': see *The Complete Works of Aristotle*, p. 736. (We

will return to the subject of apparently 'trifling' matters concerning sleep later on in this chapter, through a close reading of Freud.) Aristotle's argument here seems to chime with Bergson's notion that what we experience in dreams is 'the entire mental life minus the effort of concentration'.

5 Maurice Blanchot, *The Space of Literature*, trans. Ann Smock (Lincoln & London: University of Nebraska Press, 1989), p. 265.

6 As I say, Blanchot risks looking overly hasty in his brief and somewhat undeveloped reference to Bergson here. For Bergson, perception – whether in dreams or waking life – is only a particular and derivative filtering of the image-Real that produces a subject. In whatever state, awake or asleep, the brain is just this filtering or 'framing' process, and thus it may be construed as an image which condenses other images. (In this regard, oddly enough, one might trace certain affinities between Bergson and Blanchot around a thinking of the image, a thinking on Blanchot's part that is in fact developed in Herschel Farbman's *The Other Night*, to which I refer on a number of occasions in this book.) Hence, what strikes Bergson as the starting point of enquiry is not the submerged return of the past as dream-image while asleep, but the fact that the past is not before us in its entirety while we are awake, for this past is actually simply the Real of imagery that goes to make up everything. From this account, Bergson is assuredly not a subject-centred thinker (Blanchot leaves open such a suggestion to the non-reader of Bergson by implying that Bergson's conception of sleep is, effectively, day-oriented, and that the inattention to the world during sleep of which Bergson speaks in fact 'conserves us for the world and affirms the world'). Bergson holds on to consciousness qua affect or sensation, but it is not anthropomorphic for him, and more a kind of movement (he uses the term 'psychics' as the opposite in movement to 'physics'), so that ultimately the subject is derivative and must be transcended. I am most grateful to John Mullarkey for helping me with these ideas.

7 Sigmund Freud, *The Interpretation of Dreams*, trans. Joyce Crick (Oxford: Oxford University Press, 2008). Further page references will be given in the body of the chapter.

8 Sigmund Freud, *Jokes and Their Relation to the Unconscious*, in *The Standard Edition of the Complete Psychological Works*, Vol. VIII, ed. and trans. James Strachey (London: Hogarth Press, 1960), pp. 3–248. Further page references will be given in the body of the chapter.

9 As Freud's writing develops, he is increasingly keen to point out that what characterizes sleep is that it involves a certain relaxation of resistances to unconscious material, and is thus a precondition for the construction or

formation of dreams; nonetheless, he repeatedly insists that sleep does not
entirely quell the capacity to repress or censor the content of the dream, so that
dreams emerge as a compromise-formation in relation to psychic life in general.
Indeed, in *The Interpretation of Dreams*, Freud had argued that '*the state of sleep
makes the formation of dreams possible by reducing the endopsychic censorship*' (p.
342); yet he also associated the state of sleep with a 'suppression of affects', the
complex effect of which nonetheless had to do with the persistence of censorship,
which Freud saw as an integral part of the compromise that is produced by a
conflict between psychic forces while dreaming (p. 305).

10 Indeed, in the *Interpretation of Dreams* Freud had spoken of the Preconscious
   – and indeed the 'dominant system' – in terms of '*wish to sleep*' (p. 373), while,
   much later on in his career, he was to reiterate that 'the sleeping ego ... is focused
   on the wish to maintain sleep', overcoming potential disturbances to sleep by
   translating them, via dreams, into the 'harmless *fulfilment of a wish*' (See 'An
   Outline of Psycho-Analysis', in *The Standard Edition*, Vol. XXIII (London:
   Hogarth Press, 1964), p. 170).

11 Much later in his career, in 'An Autobiographical Study' (*The Standard Edition*,
   Vol. XX (London: Hogarth Press, 1964), pp. 7-70), Freud writes that 'dreams are
   constructed like a neurotic symptom: they are compromises between the demands
   of a repressed impulse and the resistance of a censoring force in the ego ... the
   general function of dreaming ... serves the purpose of fending off, by a kind
   of soothing action, external or internal stimuli which would tend to arouse the
   sleeper, and thus of securing sleep against interruption' (p. 45). (As Freud states
   elsewhere, it is as the expression of a compromise that the dream provides a key to
   its own interpretation; furthermore, just the type of compromise that the dream
   represents provides the grounds to interpret all manner of neurosis and psychosis
   in waking life.) Later still, in 'Revision of the Theory of Dreams' (*The Standard
   Edition*, Vol. XXII (London: Hogarth Press, 1964), pp. 7–30), Freud will insist
   once more that it is the 'unconscious impulse' that is the 'true creator of the dream'
   (p. 19) – although, of course, dreaming and sleep are not the same thing, as he
   elsewhere asserts; and sleep itself has only a partial duty, as it were, to the system of
   the unconscious, having also a clear tie to the concerns of the day (notably, serving
   the interests of rest). Indeed, here, Freud nevertheless continues as follows: 'the
   dream ... is already a compromise-structure. It has a double function; on the one
   hand, it is ego-syntonic, since, by getting rid of the stimuli which are interfering
   with sleep, it serves the wish to sleep; on the other hand it allows a repressed
   instinctual impulse to obtain the satisfaction that is possible in these circumstances,
   in the form of the hallucinated fulfilment of a wish' (p. 19). In Part 1 of 'An Outline

of Psycho-Analysis', meanwhile, Freud writes that 'dreams may arise either from the id or from the ego', since they may express an unconscious wish which 'finds enough strength during sleep to make itself felt by the ego' (p. 166) or they may communicate 'an urge left over from waking life, a preconscious train of thought' which is reinforced by an 'unconscious element' during sleep. Interestingly, some years later than the text in question, in *Beyond the Pleasure Principle* (*The Standard Edition*, Vol. XVIII (London: Hogarth Press, 1957), pp. 7–66), Freud finds himself in the midst of a discussion of certain kinds of dreams which cannot be made to fit in with the idea of dreaming as essentially about wish-fulfilment. Here, he is led to conclude that 'the function of dreams, which consists in setting aside any motives which might interrupt sleep, by fulfilling the wishes of the disturbing impulses, is not their *original* function' (p. 33). While a consideration of those exceptions to the rule of wish-fulfilment culminate in this proposition, it is Freud's argument about the temporality of the pleasure principle that leads to his suggestion that 'there was also a time before the purpose of dreams was the fulfilment of wishes' (p. 33). Nonetheless, the very statement that 'the function of dreams' is not in fact 'their *original* function' may be of interest in relation to the argument about auto-immunity I will go on to develop in this chapter.

12 Sigmund Freud, 'On Narcissism', in *The Standard Edition*, Vol. XIV (London: Hogarth Press, 1957), pp. 73–104. Further page references will be given in the body of the chapter.

13 Sigmund Freud, 'A Metapsychological Supplement to the Theory of Dreams', in *The Standard Edition*, Vol. XIV (London: Hogarth Press, 1957), pp. 222–36. Further page references will be given in the body of the chapter.

14 While this standpoint begins to unravel during the essay in question, as Freud's argument about the fundamental narcissism of sleep runs aground of the psychoanalytic logic he wishes to develop, nevertheless it is also apparent in other essays, for instance 'Thoughts for the Times on War and Death' (*The Standard Edition*, Vol. XIV (London: Hogarth Press, 1957), pp. 273–300), where Freud observes that 'all our dreams are governed by purely egoistic motives' (p. 286) – to which, in fact, Strachey appends a note stating that 'Freud later qualified this view in an addition made in 1925 to a footnote to *The Interpretation of Dreams*'; a qualification, albeit on the strength of the very same anecdote Freud tells in 'Thoughts for the Times on War and Death' which concerns the reply by an American lady to Ernest Jones, in which she insisted on the basic altruism (rather than the egoism) of her compatriots' dreams.

15 We should note here that in 'The Libido Theory and Narcissism' (*The Standard Edition*, Vol. XVI (London: Hogarth Press, 1963), pp. 412–30), Freud somewhat

distinguishes narcissism and egoism on the grounds that narcissism 'is the libidinal complement to egoism. When we speak of egoism, we have in view only the individual's *advantage*; when we talk of narcissism we are also taking his libidinal satisfaction into account' (p. 417). This distinction between narcissism and egoism is not just a static one, however, but relates to a complex interplay of forces within psychic life in its entirety.

16 Freud elsewhere insists that he will 'invariably try to separate libido from interest', or, put differently, 'the sexual and the self-preservation instincts' (see 'The Libido Theory and Narcissism', p. 420), although in 'A Metapsychological Supplement to the Theory of Dreams' the reference to 'libidinal or other interest' may be not so much a lapse as a more substantive feature of a certain deconstructibility that is working itself out in this text. Nevertheless, in 'The Libido Theory and Narcissism' Freud upholds the merits of this distinction on the grounds of the development of his thought. In any event, here he states that the libido never acquires 'egoistic interest' (p. 420), presumably leaving open the question at this point in his writing of whether it has any 'interest' at all, and of what kind.

17 In this same essay, Freud implies that dreams safeguard our slumber by dealing with possible interruptions to sleep from various external stimuli, but also that they maintain sleep by projecting an 'internal demand' onto 'an external experience, whose demand has been disposed of' (p. 223) – a visualized memory, perhaps, or an image or sequence of images now divested of the intrinsic capacity to excite fundamental concern. This defence mechanism, then, involves the substitution of a concern that can be overcome for one that cannot, precisely because the 'internal instinctual claim' (as Freud puts it) remains deeply unresolved, while the 'external danger' brought to mind in the dream has in effect already been reconciled (p. 224). Here, once more, we have a double movement whereby the dream that defends against worldly stimuli also provokes 'external experience' in order to preserve sleep, not just protecting interiority against the outside from which it withdraws, but also forcefully projecting internal concerns onto the screen of exterior life in the interests of the same outcome: sleep itself. Since the 'external experience' is reactivated precisely on the strength that it somehow translates an 'internal demand' (albeit in disempowering fashion), the narcissistic dream – the narcissism of the dream – complicates itself to the extent that it defends against what it also provokes, therefore defending against itself.

18 It is also worth noting, in this context, that in his closing comments to 'A Metapsychological Supplement to the Theory of Dreams', Freud writes that dreams as 'a residue of mental activity' are 'made possible by the fact that the narcissistic state of sleep has not been able to be completely established' (p. 234).

19 It is interesting that in *Studies on Hysteria* (*The Standard Edition*, Vol. II (London: Hogarth Press, 1957)), written during the 1890s, Breuer effectively dismisses sleep from psychological enquiry by implying that it is of a purely 'physical basis' (p. 192). Breuer suggests that, since it unquestionably represents a 'state of total unconsciousness', the deepest sleep – dreamless sleep, or sleep 'proper' – remains utterly unreceptive to psychological science. For Breuer, slumber is characterized by the minimization of 'excitation' that typifies waking or psychical life. He explains awakening unprovoked by external stimuli as the result of the accumulation of unspent or surplus energy – or, to be more precise, the non-conversion of 'tensile force into live energy' – which becomes burdensome and unpleasant, prompting a need to wake and thus transform this dormant force into functioning energy. Hence, from its earliest times we can still trace a tendency within psychoanalytic thought to sideline sleep as purely physiological (that is, outside the life of the 'mind'), and indeed to treat any form of awakening not prompted by the stimulation of the 'mind' as just a type of physical effect (even though 'excitation' is here used to describe waking life itself, and yet also to explain why sleep cannot bear itself indefinitely).

20 It is worth noting here that in 'Revision of The Theory of Dreams', Freud writes: 'For let us bear firmly in mind that, as was already pointed out by Aristotle, dream-life is the way in which our mind works during the state of sleep' (p. 16), thus connecting psychoanalysis with a whole tradition that sees sleep as a physiological platform for concerns that are predominantly those of the *mind*, consciousness, sense-perception, etc.

21 In her essay, 'On Not Being Able to Sleep' (which this chapter goes on to discuss as some length), Jacqueline Rose notes that in a letter to Fliess from 1899 Freud 'self-disparagingly dismisses his conviction that the dream is the guardian of sleep' as merely a generalization, a 'platitude' or 'commonplace' (p. 113). 'By the time of *An Outline of Psycho-Analysis*', writes Rose, 'he has qualified it: "a dream is invariably an *attempt* to get rid of a disturbance of sleep [...] The attempt may succeed more or less completely: it may also fail"' (cited in Rose, p. 113). Rose goes on to uncover other moments in Freud's text where sleep is foregone or renounced because of the fear of dreams.

22 Many years later, in 'My Contact with Josef Popper-Lynkeus' (*The Standard Edition*, Vol. XXII (London: Hogarth Press, 1964), pp. 219–26), Freud writes, starkly: 'it may be that the unconscious never sleeps at all' (p. 222).

23 Jacqueline Rose, 'On Not Being Able to Sleep: Rereading *The Interpretation of Dreams*', in *On Not Being Able to Sleep: Psychoanalysis and the Modern World* (London: Chatto and Windus, 2003), pp. 105–24. Further page references will be given in the body of the chapter.

24 Rose speculates that this understanding of psychoanalysis might dramatically change both its teaching in university humanities departments and its future among disciples and practitioners.

25 Jean-Luc Nancy, *The Fall of Sleep* (New York: Fordham University Press, 2009), p. 8.

26 As Rose notes, Freud acknowledges that the ego sleeps, and wishes for sleep, yet he insists that it remains active and alert in its role concerning dream-censorship.

Chapter 3

1 Nicolas de Warren, 'The Inner Night: Towards a Phenomenology of (Dreamless) Sleep', in *Phaenomenologica* 97: *On Time: New Contributions to the Husserlian Phenomenology of Time* (2010), pp. 273–94. Further page references will be given in the body of the chapter.

2 Maurice Merleau-Ponty, *Phenomenology of Perception*, trans. Colin Smith (London: Routledge and Kegan Paul, 1962), p. 168. Further page references will be given in the body of the chapter.

3 In several places throughout this book, I discuss the complexities concerning what Jean-Luc Nancy has called the 'conscious plunge of consciousness into unconsciousness' (see Nancy's *The Fall of Sleep*, p. 8).

4 *Not*, that is, the royal road to the 'unconscious'.

Chapter 4

1 Paul Celan, 'Edgar Jené and The Dream About The Dream' in *Collected Prose*, trans. Rosemarie Waldrop (Manchester: Carcanet, 1999), pp. 3–10. Page references will be given in the body of the chapter.

2 See Jacques Derrida, 'Shibboleth: For Paul Celan', in *Sovereignties in Question: The Poetics of Paul Celan*, (eds) Thomas Dutoit and Outi Pasanen (New York: Fordham University Press, 2005), pp. 1–64.

3 In fact the text closes with the suggestion that we now 'try to make pledges in our sleep' (p. 10), pledges that differ from the 'many oaths' that 'we have sworn in our waking lives' (p. 9): sleep-pledges that are not, therefore, made 'in the hot shadow of impatient flags, backlighted by an alien death, at the high altar of our sanctified reason' (p. 9). The pledges made during sleep lead, instead, to the ascent – indeed the creation – of an extraordinary tower, 'our face breaking through at the top' (a 'clenched stone face'), although not yet at the top, with the climb – the 'way'

– still somewhat ahead (p. 10). 'Taller than ourselves', we are able to 'look down on ourselves', and to swear our oaths, to see ourselves turned into 'a clenched fist, a fist of eyes swearing', as we become 'a thousand times ourselves, a great, overwhelming force'. And if we promise ourselves 'to tomorrow's truth', this entails a pledge that 'we do not know yet'. First appearing in 1948, written by a Jewish survivor, this ending obviously invites a certain interpretation, some of the implications of which perhaps make for less comfortable reading with the hindsight of more than 60 years. However, it is worth underlining that the 'pledges in our sleep' of which Celan speaks are set firmly against those of 'our waking lives' (p. 9) – not just those of 'reason', but also (and no doubt relatedly) those linked to the blind allegiance of the masses, to flag-waving, warfare, and 'alien death'. Moreover, the elevation of a body that is multiplied a thousand times, and headed by a 'clenched stone face', still results in a gaze, a vision, that has not yet caught up with itself, and yet which has already outrun itself; and a 'face' that envisages pledges which, at the same time, it cannot possibly foresee or, therefore, dominate. If the future is to be rebuilt by this apparently composite body, face and gaze, it therefore remains – constitutively – a dislocated body, a dreamt body that is also impossibly surreal; as dislocated and impossibly surreal, perhaps, as the myriad figures which emerge throughout the dream 'about' the dream. The tower that rises up, the thousand-strong face, 'a clenched fist, a fist of eyes swearing', promising what it cannot yet know – this is perhaps an anxious if not a frightening prospect for many a contemporary reader; but, equally, we should not overlook the fact that it also presents a highly complex and irreducible image, notably in the context of Celan's essay and his writing overall.

Chapter 5

1 Jacques Derrida, 'Living On/Borderlines', in *Deconstruction and Criticism*, Harold Bloom et al. (London and Henley: Routledge and Kegan Paul, 1979), pp. 75–176. Further page references will be given in the body of the chapter.

2 Jacques Derrida, 'The Double Session', in *Dissemination*, trans. Barbara Johnson (Chicago: Chicago University Press, 1981) pp. 187–316.

3 Jacques Derrida, 'Letter to a Japanese Friend', in *Psyche: Inventions of the Other, Volume II*, (eds) Peggy Kamuf and Elizabeth Rottenberg (Stanford: Stanford University Press, 2008), pp. 1–6.

4 See Giorgio Agamben, *The End of the Poem: Studies in Poetics*, trans. Daniel Heller-Roazen (Stanford: Stanford University Press, 1999).

5 Jacques Derrida, 'Shibboleth', in *Sovereignties in Question: The Poetics of Paul Celan*, eds Thomas Dutoit and Outi Pasanen (New York: Fordham University Press, 2005), pp. 1–64. Further page references will be given in the body of the chapter.

6 Jacques Derrida, 'Che cos'è la poesia?', in *A Derrida Reader: Between the Blinds*, ed. Peggy Kamuf (New York: Columbia University Press, 1991), pp. 221–40.

7 Maurice Blanchot, *L'Arrêt de mort/Death Sentence*, trans. Lydia Davis (Barrytown, NY: Station Hill, 1998). Further page references will be given in the body of the chapter.

8 Maurice Blanchot, 'Dreaming, Writing', in *Friendship*, trans. Elizabeth Rottenberg (Stanford: Stanford University Press, 1997), pp. 140–8. Further page references will be given in the body of the chapter.

9 In 'Dreaming, Writing', the desire to recount the dream lies behind several kinds of address to the other, constituting 'an obscure need' to make our dreams 'more real by living with someone else the singularity that belongs to them and would seem to address one person alone'. This, perhaps draws us 'close to literature', says Blanchot, 'at least to its enigmas, its glamour, its illusions' – although, via Leiris, he is quick to characterize the 'exactness' of the relation between dreaming and writing in terms of the literary affirmation of 'poetic signs' which constitute the dream, or from which it emerges, rather than taking dreams more simply as the expression of psychoanalytic or autobiographical 'truth' (pp. 142–3).

10 Maurice Blanchot, 'In the Night That Is Watched Over', in *Political Writings, 1953-1993*, trans. Zakir Paul (New York: Fordham University Press, 2010), p. 133.

11 Maurice Blanchot, *The Writing of the Disaster*, trans. Ann Smock (Lincoln & London: University of Nebraska Press, 1995). Further page references will be given in the body of the chapter.

12 Maurice Blanchot, *The Space of Literature*, trans. Ann Smock (Lincoln & London: University of Nebraska Press, 1989), pp. 264–8. Further page references will be given in the body of the chapter.

13 Maurice Blanchot, *The Infinite Conversation*, trans. Susan Hanson (Minneapolis: University of Minnesota Press, 1993), p. 385.

14 Writing of Kafka's *The Burrow*, Blanchot remarks in *The Space of Literature*: 'to construct the burrow is to open night to the *other* night'. For Blanchot, to seek the 'bad' intimacy of pure self-enclosure in the total repose of sleep is in fact to expose oneself to the dreams which, beyond the limits of self-control, inevitably expose one to the 'outside' – since otherwise total separation would lead to the fatal demise of the very same self in question, a self seeking to defend itself absolutely. To 'burrow' in or 'burrow' down is therefore to expose the self to the limits of itself, the outside *of* itself in the 'other night' (p. 169).

15 According to a certain line of thinking in philosophy, of course, death happens to 'no-one' in the sense that the subject by definition cannot experience their own death.

16 Emmanuel Levinas, *Time and the Other*, trans. Richard A. Cohen (Pittsburgh, PA: Duquesne University Press, 1987). Further page references will be given in the body of the chapter.

17 Emmanuel Levinas, *Existence and Existents*, trans. Alphonso Lingis (Pittsburgh, Pennsylvania: Duquesne University Press, 2001). Further page references will be given in the body of the chapter.

18 Robert Bernasconi, Foreword to Levinas's *Existence and Existents*, trans. Alphonso Lingis, pp. vii–xv. See p. xii. Further page references will be given in the body of the chapter.

19 Emmanuel Levinas, 'God and Philosophy', in *Collected Philosophical Papers*, trans. Alphonso Lingis (Pittsburgh, PA: Duquesne University Press, 1998), pp. 153–73. Further page references will be given in the body of the chapter.

Chapter 6

1 Samuel Beckett, *Cascando*, in *The Complete Dramatic Works* (London: Faber and Faber, 1986), pp. 295–304. Further references will be given in the body of the chapter.

2 Samuel Beckett, *Company*, in *Nohow On* (New York: Grove Press, 1996), pp. 1–46. Further references will be given in the body of the chapter.

3 Alain Badiou, *On Beckett* (Manchester: Clinamen, 2003), pp. 11–13. Further references will be given in the body of the chapter.

4 John Pilling, *Samuel Beckett* (London: Routledge and Kegan Paul, 1976), p. 111. Further references will be given in the body of the chapter.

5 Michel Foucault, 'My Body, This Paper, This Fire', in *Michel Foucault, Essential Works Volume 2, 1954-1984: Aesthetics, Method, and Epistemology*, ed. James Faubion (London: Penguin Books, 1998), p. 410. In the next chapter we will explore this essay more closely, since it constitutes Foucault's response to Derrida's critique of *Madness and Civilization* (found in Derrida's essay, 'Cogito and the History of Madness'), which revolves around a contested reading of Descartes.

6 I will refer here to René Descartes, *Meditations and Other Philosophical Writings* (London: Penguin, 1998). Further references will be given in the body of the chapter.

7 Peter Boxall, *Since Beckett: Contemporary Writing in the Wake of Modernism* (New York and London: Continuum, 2009), p. 307.

Chapter 7

1 Jacques Derrida, 'Cogito and the History of Madness', in *Writing and Difference*, trans. Alan Bass (London: Routledge, 1995), pp. 31–63. Further page references will be given in the body of the chapter.

2 In the process of identifying madness with this historical age, Derrida asks whether Foucault neglects the critically important influence of the ancient and specifically Greek tradition. Derrida underlines the suggestion he finds in Foucault, that this tradition should be somewhat discounted from the history the latter wants to tell, since, as Foucault himself tells us, its 'Logos had no contrary' (cited in Derrida, p. 39). Derrida, meanwhile, speaks of 'a reason divided against itself since the dawn of its Greek origin' (p. 40).

3 It is perhaps worth noting here that the philosophical question of whether we can know if our perception or experience is indeed grounded in conscious, waking life is far from novel. For instance, although the discussion leads off in a somewhat different direction, Socrates famously asks Theaetetus what evidence he can offer that in the present instance the two men are awake, or whether it might be possible that they are asleep and dreaming in all their thoughts and conversation. See 'Theaetetus', 158b–c, in Plato, *Complete Works*, ed. John M. Cooper (Indianapolis: Hackett Publishing, 1997), p. 176.

4 In his response to Derrida, Foucault is at great pains to insist that he never claimed such a conceptual determination of madness could or should be discerned in the 'text' of Descartes.

5 Michel Foucault, 'My Body, This Paper, This Fire', in *Michel Foucault, Essential Works Volume 2, 1954-1984: Aesthetics, Method, and Epistemology*, ed. James Faubion (London: Penguin Books, 1998). Further page references will be given in the body of the chapter.

6 Jacques Derrida, '"To Do Justice to Freud": The History of Madness in the Age of Psychoanalysis', in *Resistances of Psychoanalysis*, trans. Peggy Kamuf, Pascale–Anne Brault, and Michael Naas (Stanford: Stanford University Press, 1998), pp. 70–118.

Chapter 8

1 Jean-Luc Nancy, *The Fall of Sleep* (New York, Fordham University Press, 2009). All further page references will be given in the body of the chapter.

2 Nancy quotes from Jacques Derrida, *Glas*, trans. John P. Leavey, Jr., and Richard Rand (Lincoln: University of Nebraska Press, 1986), p. 132.

3 These endorsements which appear on the back jacket of the English translation of Nancy's book are by Kevin Hart, Charles Shepherdson, and Gerald L. Bruns, respectively.

4 Indeed, this reaction to somnambulance on Nancy's part may perhaps be attributed to the Hegelian influence that runs throughout *The Fall of Sleep*. In Hegel's *Philosophy of Mind*, it is asserted that: 'The only way in which the animal organism in sleep is still related to the external world is breathing, this wholly abstract relationship to the undifferentiated element of air. With particularized externality by contrast the healthy human organism in sleep no longer stands in any relation. If, therefore, a man in sleep becomes active outwardly, then he is ill. This occurs in sleep-walkers' (G. W. F. Hegel, *Philosophy of Mind*, trans. W. Wallace and A. V. Miller (Oxford: Oxford University Press, 2007), p. 65).

5 In many of the crucial passages in *The Fall of Sleep*, Nancy can be found drawing upon Hegel, who writes: 'as sleep is the state of the soul's undifferentiatedness, so night obscures the difference between things; and as awaking displays the soul's distinguishing-itself-from-itself, so the light of day lets the differences of things emerge' (G. W. F. Hegel, *Philosophy of Mind*, p. 64).

6 Maurice Blanchot, *L'Arrêt de mort/Death Sentence*, trans. Lydia Davis (Barrytown, NY: Station Hill, 1998), p. 20.

7 Throughout *The Fall of Sleep*, sleep is taken to mark the limit of phenomenology. The dissolution or suspension of the self during slumber links the sleeper to the Kantian thing in-itself: 'The sleeping *self* does not appear: it is not phenomenalized … There is no phenomenology of sleep', and thus the sleeping self is 'self in the sense of the *thing in itself* that Kant made famous' (pp. 13–14). Thus, in sleep 'more than anything I myself become indistinct. I no longer properly distinguish myself from the world or from others, from my own body or from my own mind, either. For I can no longer hold anything as an object, as a perception or a thought, without this very thing making itself felt as being *at the same time* myself and something other than myself' (p. 7).

8 Equally, perhaps, one might recall here the wish for sleep in the Freudian preconscious.

9 The reference here is to G. W. F. Hegel, *Hegel's Philosophy of Mind: Part Three of the Encyclopaedia of the Philosophical Sciences*, trans. William Wallace (Oxford: Oxford University Press, 1971), p. 67. Nancy slightly modifies the translation. See my more detailed reading, earlier in this book, which explores the surrounding passages in Hegel in a somewhat different way than Nancy, and suggests his treatment of this quotation may not be satisfactory.

10 Jacques Derrida, 'Violence and Metaphysics: An Essay on the Thought of Emmanuel Levinas', in *Writing and Difference*, trans. Alan Bass (London: Routledge, 1995), pp. 79–153. Further page references will be given in the body of the chapter.

Bibliography

Agamben, Giorgio, *Infancy and History: On the Destruction of Experience*, trans. Liz Heron (London: Verso, 1993)

—*The End of the Poem: Studies in Poetics*, trans. Daniel Heller-Roazen (Stanford: Stanford University Press, 1999a)

—*The Man Without Content*, trans. Georgia Albert (Stanford: Stanford University Press, 1999b)

Aristotle, *The Complete Works of Aristotle, The Revised Oxford Translation*, Vol. I, ed. Jonathan Barnes (Princeton: Princeton University Press, 1984)

Badiou, Alain, *On Beckett* (Manchester: Clinamen, 2003)

Beckett, Samuel, *The Complete Dramatic Works* (London: Faber and Faber, 1986)

—*Nohow On* (New York: Grove Press, 1996)

Bergson, Henri, *Creative Evolution*, trans. Arthur Mitchell (Modern Library, Random House, 1944)

—*Mind-Energy*, trans. H. Wildon Carr, (eds) Keith Ansell Pearson and Michael Kolkman (London: Palgrave Macmillan, 2007)

Bernasconi, Robert, 'Foreword to Emmanuel Levinas', in *Existence and Existents*, trans. Alphonso Lingis (Pittsburgh: Duquesne University Press, 2001), pp. vii–xv.

Blanchot, Maurice, *The Space of Literature*, trans. Ann Smock (Lincoln and London: University of Nebraska Press, 1989)

—*The Infinite Conversation*, trans. Susan Hanson (Minneapolis: University of Minnesota Press, 1993)

—*The Writing of the Disaster*, trans. Ann Smock (Lincoln and London: University of Nebraska Press, 1995)

—*Friendship*, trans. Elizabeth Rottenberg (Stanford: Stanford University Press, 1997)

—*L'Arrêt de mort/Death Sentence*, trans. Lydia Davis (Barrytown: Station Hill, 1998)

—*Political Writings, 1953–1993*, trans. Zakir Paul (New York: Fordham University Press, 2010)

Boxall, Peter, *Since Beckett: Contemporary Writing in the Wake of Modernism* (New York and London: Continuum, 2009) de Warren, Nicolas, 'The Inner Night: Towards a Phenomenology of (Dreamless) Sleep', in *Phaenomenologica 97: On Time: New Contributions to the Husserlian Phenomenology of Time* (2010), pp. 273–94.

Derrida, Jacques, 'Living On/Borderlines', in *Deconstruction and Criticism*, (eds) Harold Bloom et al. (London and Henley: Routledge and Kegan Paul, 1979), pp. 75–176.

—*Dissemination*, trans. Barbara Johnson (Chicago: Chicago University Press, 1981)

—*Glas*, trans. John P. Leavey, Jr., and Richard Rand (Lincoln and London: University of Nebraska Press, 1986)

—*A Derrida Reader: Between the Blinds*, ed. Peggy Kamuf (New York: Columbia University Press, 1991)

—*Writing and Difference*, trans. Alan Bass (London: Routledge, 1995)

—*Resistances of Psychoanalysis*, trans. Peggy Kamuf, Pascale-Anne Brault, and Michael Naas (Stanford: Stanford University Press, 1998)

—*Sovereignties in Question: The Poetics of Paul Celan*, (eds) Thomas Dutoit and Outi Pasanen (New York: Fordham University Press, 2005)

—*Psyche: Inventions of the Other*, Volume II, (eds) Peggy Kamuf and Elizabeth Rottenberg (Stanford: Stanford University Press, 2008a)

—*The Animal That Therefore I Am*, ed. Marie-Louise Mallet, trans. David Wills (New York: Fordham University Press, 2008b)

Descartes, René, *Meditations and Other Philosophical Writings* (London: Penguin, 1998)

Ekirch, A. Roger, *At Day's Close: Night in Times Past* (New York and London: Norton, 2005)

Farbman, Herschel, *The Other Night: Dreaming, Writing, and Restlessness in Twentieth-Century Literature* (New York: Fordham University Press, 2008)

Foucault, *Essential Works Volume 2, 1954-1984: Aesthetics, Method, and Epistemology*, ed. James Faubion (London: Penguin Books, 1998)

Freud, Sigmund, *The Standard Edition of the Complete Psychological Works* in 24 vols., ed. and trans. James Strachey (London: Hogarth Press, 1956–74)

—*The Interpretation of Dreams*, trans. Joyce Crick (Oxford: Oxford University Press, 2008)

Hegel, G. W. F., *Philosophy of Mind*, trans. W. Wallace and A. V. Miller (Oxford: Oxford University Press, 2007)

Heidegger, Martin, *Being and Time*, trans. John Macquarie and Edward Robinson (New York: Harper and Row, 1962)

Hobson, J. Allan, *Dreaming: An Introduction to the Science of Sleep* (Oxford: Oxford University Press, 2002)

Horne, Jim, *Sleepfaring: A Journey through the Science of Sleep* (Oxford: Oxford University Press, 2006)

Kant, Immanuel, *Anthropology, History and Education (The Cambridge Edition of the Works of Immanuel Kant)*, (eds) Günter Zöller and Robert B. Londen (Cambridge: Cambridge University Press, 2007)

Levinas, Emmanuel, *Time and the Other*, trans. Richard A. Cohen (Pittsburgh: Duquesne University Press, 1987)

—*Collected Philosophical Papers*, trans. Alphonso Lingis (Pittsburgh: Duquesne University Press, 1998)

—*Existence and Existents*, trans. Alphonso Lingis (Pittsburgh: Duquesne University Press, 2001)

Meddis, Ray, *The Sleep Instinct* (London: Routledge and Kegan Paul, 1977)

Merleau-Ponty, Maurice, *Phenomenology of Perception*, trans. Colin Smith (London: Routledge and Kegan Paul, 1962)

Nancy, Jean-Luc, *The Fall of Sleep* (New York: Fordham University Press, 2009)

Pilling, John, *Samuel Beckett* (London: Routledge and Kegan Paul, 1976)

Plato, *The Collected Dialogues*, (eds) Edith Hamilton and Huntingdon Cairns (Princeton: Princeton University Press, 1961)

—*Complete Works*, ed. John M. Cooper (Indianapolis: Hackett Publishing, 1977)

Rose, Jacqueline, *On Not Being Able to Sleep: Psychoanalysis and the Modern World* (London: Chatto and Windus, 2003)

Stickgold, Robert and Matthew P. Walker, (eds) *The Neuroscience of Sleep*, (Burlington: Academic Press, 2009)

Watkin, William, *The Literary Agamben: Adventures in Logopoiesis* (London and New York: Continuum, 2010)

Weber, Samuel, *Benjamin's –abilities* (Cambridge, MA., and London: Harvard University Press, 2008)

Williams, Simon J., *The Politics of Sleep: Governing (Un)consciousness in the Late Modern Age* (Basingstoke: Palgrave Macmillan, 2011)

Index